Without A Village

A modern day look at mothering in a broken system and how to get through it

REBECCA PIERCE

Rebecca Pierce
BOOKS

Without a Village Copyright ©2023 by Rebecca Pierce

All rights reserved. No part of this book may be used or reproduced in any manner whatsoever without the permission of the author except in the case of brief quotations embodied in articles or critical reviews. For Information, address contact@rebeccapiercebooks.com

While the author has made every effort to provide accurate information at the time of writing and publication, neither the publisher nor the author assumes any responsibility for errors or for changes that occur after publication and hereby disclaims any liability to any party for any loss, damage, or disruption caused by errors or omissions, whether such errors or omissions result from negligence, accident, or any other cause.

The publisher and the author make no guarantees concerning the level of success you may experience by following the advice and strategies contained in this book, and you accept the risk that results will differ for each individual.

Names have been changed where personal stories are discussed to protect the identity of the individuals.

Some sample scenarios in this book are fictitious. Any similarity to actual persons, living or dead, is coincidental.

FIRST EDITION

Cover Illustration by: Lea Androić

Library of Congress Cataloging-in-Publication Data has been applied for

ISBN:
978-1-7390111-1-6 (ebook)
978-1-7390111-0-9 (Paperback)
978-1-7390111-2-3 (Hardcover)

DEDICATION

To my husband Kyle, who went through a transformational shift from the start of our parenthood journey to now. It could have ended in divorce and resentment–i'm happy it didn't.

And to my children...
It's not you.

You are the greatest gift the world has ever given me. I hope you grow up in a society that realizes raising children should not be an inconvenience, a prison sentence, or an act of courage. I will support you and your children, and I will always fight for a system that holds itself accountable for the struggles of motherhood.

CONTENTS

Introduction vii

Chapter 1   A Brief History of Motherhood 1
    The 1800s: When Things Started to Change 1
    A Shift in the 1960s Through the 1980s 5
    Today's Mom 9
    Fed Up 13

Chapter 2   The Invisible Woman 18
    Inherent Gender Bias 18
    Identity Loss 25

Chapter 3   The Default Parent 36
    How Women Became the Default Parent 42

Chapter 4   The Pressures of Motherhood 49
    The Myth of Motherhood 49
    Sacrifices Made 54

Chapter 5   Sharing the Load 60
    10 Tips on Sharing the Physical Load 64
    10 Tips on Sharing the Mental Load 76
    10 Practical Tips for Single Moms 90

Chapter 6 Build Your Confidence 104
- Join the Confidence Era 106

Chapter 7 Take Care of *You* First 129
- Why Self-Care Is Vital for Motherhood.................................... 129
- Physical Self-Care... 131
- Mental Self-Care.. 139
- Social Self-Care.. 152

Chapter 8 Get Out of Your Head 158
- Negative Mind, Negative Life 158
- Overthinking and Its Effects on Motherhood 160
- Understand Your Thought Patterns 164
- Change Your Thinking.. 175

Chapter 9 Creating Your Mom-ifesto 185
- The What and Why of a Personal Manifesto 185
- Write a Personal Mom-ifesto 187

Chapter 10 Journaling as Therapy 194
- How Journaling Will Benefit You and Your Children 196
- Journal Prompts to Get You Started 198

Conclusion... 201
Acknowledgments.. 206
References.. 208

INTRODUCTION

> You are exactly the mother that your child needs, knowing that will change your entire perspective on motherhood.
> —LAUREN TINGLEY

I remember my little boy's first year vividly as a beautiful grey period. When he was born, the sun inside me lit up like it had never shone before, but it also found a way to at the same time, be engulfed in a never-ending solar eclipse. It was the year that I most frequently compromised myself, mentally substituting my needs to satisfy his constant but precious demands, and subjecting myself to self-loathing because I had not yet nailed the art of motherhood.

I kept telling myself that I would get better at it. That there would come a day when I would be satisfied with the state of my apartment (that was too small for us to begin with), and also be content with my position on the long ladder of acceptable mothering requirements like looking well-rested, happy, and put together. To my dismay, time would show me, frequently and consistently, that my version of mothering somehow fell below today's criterion for the perfect mother.

When I was seconds away from exhaustion, breastfeeding my sick infant in the early hours of the morning, I was the stay-at-home mother that didn't know how to preserve her own identity in the wake of her motherhood. When I put myself through the 4am rises to prepare my husbands breakfast for the mornings of his shift work, meals for the day, and stumbled through the late-night cleaning fests that ensured our home looked presentable, I was the mother that was far too obsessed with homemaking to have time for herself, and often times for her husband too.

Regardless of what I did, motherhood only seemed to be able to exhaust me. It told me that I didn't deserve my sleep because, as a stay-at-home mother, I had to be a vision of the perfect housewife in order to make up for the fact that I lacked a *real job*. It taught me that unless I was worked to the bone, I was a lazy mother who couldn't bother to keep up with the rising trends of motherhood and feminism. It taught me that, as overstimulated and out-of-touch as I felt, I had to push myself to satisfy my child at the moment he needed me—and occasionally, my husband too if I could force myself into romance without considering how much sleep I would lose if I pushed my bedtime back another 30 minutes. Repeatedly, I found myself invested in a version of motherhood that demanded constant and thankless tasks and sacrifices that drained me of my energy and sense of humanity.

When it all got too much for me to handle, I came clean about the struggles I'd been hiding from my friends and family to a mom group that I had joined as a last resort to save my sanity in all my scepticism. To my comforting yet unfortunate surprise, I was not alone in the uphill climb of trying to become society's perfect mother. The ready exchange of ideas in conversation showed me that mothers were universally being scammed—sold the idea of reaching an impossible ideal that was out of touch with the reality that women face on a daily basis. It takes a village to raise a child, but the modern woman is expected to achieve this feat on her own while managing a career in an institutionalized society that will never recognize her worth. The model of the perfect mother is a walking contradiction—always content, even in her exhaustion, and absolutely capable, even when no parts of her day allow her some time for herself.

Realize, there is no way to live up to this false image, which will keep haunting you in its impossibility. It will simply set you up for pain.

Why is it so difficult to find the holy grail of work-life balance that everyone raves about? Is it because you are not working hard enough, or is it because this balance itself is a carefully constructed myth? Why do you feel like you cannot tell your partner that they should be doing more of their share of parenting? Is it because they are actually supporting you in the way that they need to, or because you are afraid of turning into that whiny new mom that you see complaining personified on TV?

Becoming a mom is like walking into a world that has dramatically positioned itself against you overnight. Being the antihero of your story, the world and its rules present you with impossibility. Today's version of motherhood holds you accountable for its own shortcomings. If you are a new mother and you find that you feel this way, know that you are experiencing the universal dismay of mothers who find themself duped by society's broken system for motherhood.

On both domestic and professional fronts, mothers have grown accustomed to accommodating the interests of other individuals over their own. More often than not, our goals, dreams, nutrition (and even our sanities), have been considered secondary to greater causes that often seek to satisfy the interests of politics and men. Being a mother should not be an act of self-denial. Our current cultural climate toward parenting splits a disproportionate amount of responsibility on fathers and mothers, leaving mothers to carry the brunt of its weight. The negativity that our culture has normalized toward women, regardless of their choices in occupation, has made both working and stay-at-home life uncomfortable options that a mother has to choose from. Whichever move she makes is considered to be selfish, for whichever reason society decides to condemn her with—it does not have to be this way.

As you read this book, you will be introduced to different ways in which you can care for yourself, and your mental health as a mom and as a human even on 'the difficult days'. We will also delve into a few older tricks in the universe's handbook of mothering. It is possible that my words may not provide the most accurate or faithful interpretations of your unique struggles. Motherhood, after all, is a deeply subjective experience. What I believe we can achieve together, is a progressive dialogue toward a better version of motherhood than that which we have been presented with today.

The panic of today, where your life seems to move in a flurry of diaper changes and messy feeds, will likely subside in the future. You will most definitely hold the reins and have this entire gig nailed to perfection in less time than you think. Till then, let *Without a Village* be your temporary recluse. One which you can turn to on the days that you feel like the patriarchy chewed off too much of your patience. Let these words envelop you in a realm of their own, providing you with the acceptance that our society has yet to produce.

In writing this book, I hope to present to you the ways in which motherhood can be made to be a celebratory existence– even on the days you feel completely broken. Together, we will work toward breaking the toxic ideals associated with motherhood to forge a version of the mother that is authentic to her own needs and individuality. Fortifying confidence in the wake of guilt and insecurity, let us rise as mothers who are not afraid of breaking the glass walls that have caged us.

Thank you for taking on this emotional, powerful, ugly- beautiful journey that is motherhood with me, and all the other divine mothers out there. Together, I believe we can bring back the village.

CHAPTER 1

A BRIEF HISTORY OF MOTHERHOOD

> "But behind all your stories is your mother's story, for hers is where yours begins."
> —MITCH ALBOM

The 1800s: When Things Started to Change

The changing opinions associated with women and femininity for the past century has resulted in a multitude of ways in which motherhood can be thought of. While it may not be best to glorify a past which we have gained social and economic liberation from, observing the changing cultural perspectives held toward the act of mothering may show a fascinating timeline of history that we share together—allowing us to delve into the contrasts between the mothering cultures of the past and those that we practice today.

Let's consider what it may have looked like for mothers— Imagine the year is 1849. Mary is 18 years old. She is the mother of her first child. Mary loves her little son, and can't bear to be parted from him, but raising him under her husband's leadership proves to be a task of Herculean efforts. Her husband William is as well-meaning as they come, but undeniably firm that he doesn't want his children raised by just *anybody*. There would be no mammies, or nurses for them. His children deserved every ounce of their mother's attention in being fed, changed, and looked after. All the other workers wives tended to their children like such, and the effort was bound to show. As William heads off to his long hours at the local mill, toiling away at the dust and grime that all the new machines were bringing, Mary finds herself worn thin by her efforts to tend to her child in a manner that is faithful to her husbands vision. Despite her concentrated efforts, she always seems to be falling short of being a satisfactory caretaker. Either the water in the bath becomes cold too soon, or her son refuses his breakfast, it always seems to be something. Sometimes, she finds herself considering how peaceful it would be to be free of his shrill screams and his constant need to be looked after whether happy or sad— just for an afternoon, or a few days. What would a full week look like? Would it be like burying your head in the sand, to disappear from responsibility only till your soul felt like it were fit to take it on again? She thought to herself "if only things were the way they had been when my mother was growing up". Her mother had *all* the help that she could have asked for. Her father had felt like her mother's education was not sufficient for the upbringing of his children, so he took up the frontiers of discipline and education. Washing, feeding, and clothing were handled by her mammy, who was only ever cheerful about her work. Her mother's tasks in parenting had been cuddling up with her during the day providing love, and telling her stories at nighttime. There had been all the care that a child *truly* needed and deserved and a division of work that felt a bit more manageable.

This may seem like an old wives tale but it brings to the table a story of generational change. As mothers of the 21st century, we are not new to this. Views and perspectives toward identity are bound to change with time. With it comes a transformation of cultural practices that we are familiar with and the task of acclimatizing to a version of the world that we are not particularly accustomed to. You may be familiar with this in a less gradual way if you were a mother at the start of 2019 who was rapidly thrown into parenting in the midst of a Covid crisis. The colonial era's treatment of motherhood sprang from a vastly different, even elitist, opinion toward the role of a wife and that of a woman. In the 1700s a woman was institutionally deprived of the same education that her male counterpart had the privilege of taking for granted. As a result, she was also deprived of any intellectual dialogue with the children she was to raise, as men deemed women to be too academically deficient to do so. The 1700s made the mother a manager of her household, juggling her employed help and also keeping track of her household expenses in order to support her husband. Considering the sheer size of a typical colonial home, this proved to be a feat of impressive skill and planning. I will not use these observations to sugarcoat the rampant misogyny, racism, and class gaps that the colonial times were known for though. Even when men took it upon themselves to tend to their children's education and also instill moral values upon them, there was never any record of them handling squabbling babies or dealing with blowouts. When men had been involved (to a comparatively significant degree) in the life of their children, caregiving was thought to be an act beneath them. Even as help was provided in raising the child—in the form of employed servants, slave women (dubbed "mammies," perhaps to remove the enforced labor from their titles), midwives, and other members of the household—mothering was unquestionably a feminine act.

What the 1800s and Victorian thinking of that era granted, in contrast, was the concept of a mother being a singular caretaker of her children. The social, cultural, and economic implications of the industrial revolution led to a transformative change in the way that families handled themselves, resulting in a novel form of the regular domestic division of labor that took into account the longer hours of work that men had to adhere to. As you would imagine, the spontaneous change in lifestyle clashed with the Victorian school of thought that promoted mothers to essentially be the sole caregiver. What resulted was many women being diagnosed with a case of "nervous temperament," which was unsurprisingly growing common in the mothers of the population.

Freshly postpartum, women found themselves pushed toward nine days of nonnegotiable bed rest and isolation. Even partners were prohibited from speaking to them for more than five minutes as excitement was deemed to be dangerous to their health, especially when they were in a fragile position. While many of us would adore the "me time" that everyone in the Victorian era seemed to be so obsessed with, there was more to the isolation that women were made to endure than respect for their hardships. Their period of rest was considered too delicate to be intruded on by any form of physical exertion. Books and writing were prohibited. What this left for the women was the debilitating task of being forced into purposelessness in the name of their security. This form of treatment was lengthened and even more rigidly imposed on women who were assumed to be suffering from nervous temperaments. Charlotte Perkins Gilman, the writer of the famous short story, "The Yellow Wallpaper," had been one such woman. She was subjected to this diagnosis a year after the birth of her first daughter. At the time, the most popular treatment for this condition involved enforcing "rest cure," a procedure that involved isolating patients and restricting them from all kinds of physical and mental exertions. Patients were routinely made to avoid reading, writing, and exercising—leaving them to dwell in their isolation.

Gilman's short story, which has been recognized for inspiring other authors such as Sylvia Plath and Alice Walker, had been written in response to her treatment by Dr. Silas Weir Mitchell. The story depicts a woman being subjected to rest cure and describes her feelings of being left with nothing to do but observe the old nursery room that she had been forced to inhabit. Consequently, she begins to become troubled by the room's yellow wallpaper, growing concerned that a woman is being caged within it. By the end of the story the woman, unhinged from being forced to be idle in order to cure herself, rips at the wallpaper, believing that she has freed the woman that has been caged inside it. Although a fictional account of the procedure, the struggle of the woman in the story represents the struggle of vulnerable women who had been sentenced to isolation as a form of therapy. The experiences of Gilman and these women add to the standing tradition of depriving women of their agency to voice their concerns and exercise their true needs. "The Yellow Wallpaper" proved to be revolutionary in creating progress for better preserving the rights of women in the field of mental health. Gilman's words were able to convince Mitchell to alter his treatment practice in a way that was less pervasive of their personal rights. Even if this is a story that is, by comparison, more successful than most in this era, it is truly unfortunate that it took so much pain and suffering for the women to be heard above the voices of the men who believed it best to silence them.

A Shift in the 1960s Through the 1980s

As the wheel of time took its slow turn between wars, various child-rearing practices, women's and citizen's rights revolutions, and the paperwork that came with it, we learned to reassess our lifestyles to accommodate families that would better satisfy the modernity that we found ourselves in. The Equal Pay Act of 1963 meant that the same work would promise the same wage—without sex, religion, race, or color influencing payment. Title *VII* of the Civil Rights Act of 1964 prevented workplace discrimination based on sex, color, religion, race, or worker origins. In 1971, the practice of private employers considering the existence of female applicants' preschool-aged children as a factor in justifying their rejection from employment was abolished. The 1978 Pregnancy Discrimination Act ensured that women were allowed to work while they were pregnant. Blanketed by a wealth of legal legislature to protect their rights, the rates of women turning to work were higher than ever. Daycares seemed to be on the rise—a stark contrast to how they were limited in spite of the demand for them during the war as an effort of childcare advocates who feared its detrimental effect on the typical family structure—and mothers truly seemed to be having it all.

In truth— as all forms of progress do inadvertently prove— things are never so simple. Though these changes may look like righted defaults—to the generation that witnessed them, they were spontaneous changes in the predominant form of cultural thought that had to be changed overnight. To this generation of women, who had been raised and honed to become the perfect housewives, witnessing this change in cultural thought was also witnessing a material change in need that delegated them to be without purpose. These women molded their lives based on their expected motherhood, only to be told that the system was decidedly moving past them.

What did this look like? Let's imagine of Linda, a 34 year old mother with three children. Among her favorite pastimes were 'cozying up to a good book' in the evenings, and experimenting with new dinners to surprise her husband. Her life produced a sufficient combination of work and rest for her. The year was 1960. Every television show seemed to be preoccupied with the concept of working women, and the ways that they were able to do it all. Her friend groups were growing more and more concerned about the way they led their lives. Some of them had already taken measures to go join the workforce. While Linda had supported the women's rights revolution as it went rampant on the streets, it took her great effort to swallow back some of her concerns. It was not that she didn't want women to be working. She knew enough people who deserved their rightful spots in the workforce. Still, it hurt her to see that in reinforcing the entry of 'the new woman' into existence, it was becoming increasingly shameful to be like the old woman. The change in mindset was troubling. What the television, the radio, and the newspapers seemed to be saying was not that women 'could' be working—but that they 'should' be doing so.

Why refrain from working, when you could gloat about doing it all? Worryingly though, there was no system held in place to support the working woman—especially a woman with children. Where were the kids going to stay when daycares were not exactly affordable, or readily available everywhere? While some of her friends chased the pipe dream of being career women, they were also taking on the added burden of making sure that their households were unnoticeably unaffected by their aspirations. What carefully scrubbed floors, folded laundry, and a nine-to-five job left behind, was an exhausted individual who had to handle more than they truly could. Where were the women's rights revolution and the discussion about finding fulfillment in office work when Linda's decision to raise four children had once been the peak of womanhood? In the years that she spent on home economics classes which taught her that the most correct way to be a woman was to care for her family, where were all the commercials about working women being the latest definition of a desirable woman, sexy in her capacity to balance work and household responsibilities? Where had the revolution been when her father had decided it was unnecessary for her to go to college? It was confusing...

Of course, Linda was grateful. The dramatic change made in social perspectives meant that her daughters would have a much better shot at a career than she did, but this change also meant that she would be looked down upon for a lifestyle that was not in her immediate control and one that she had grown to love. She looked at her four children and imagined herself coming home to the sudden wealth of their homework and projects that she would surely have to help them with at night. The upkeep that her household demanded would mean that her nine-to-five had to be followed by hours of chores. The personal connection she made with her children and the thousands of hugs and kisses she would miss. She considered her education and how much effort it would take her to get back on the academic horse still wanting to have it all. What stood before her was a mountain of a task that she couldn't afford to pursue, even if it qualified her to be the best version of herself. In the name of progress, women were once again pushed toward fulfilling a political fantasy that did not have the social structure that it needed to be an achievable goal for women of all classes. A system that didn't support a balance of mothering and personal fulfillment. In defaulting to 'staying at home', Linda was now considered the lazy and unproductive mother. She felt shameful because of her inability to fulfill herself. But, she was also protecting her sanity, which she valued in a new world that seemed to want to push American women to their breaking points.

What this story emphasizes is that the brand of feminism sold to women in the 60s only made itself available to women of a particular class. The working woman looked like a great concept on paper, but took a large amount of money and effort in order to become an attainable reality. This is not to disregard the milestones made in the strife that went on to bring more equality to American society. The reality that we find ourselves in today, where women have been granted a greater capability to pursue their ambitions by the systematic changes made to our shared legal legislature, cannot be overstated as the victory of the women who strove against their system in the 1900s. Acknowledging the fact that they were only backed by a support system that was only half there in facilitating them toward their goals adds a greater level of depth to their monumental achievements. By the same token, it must be realized that the new kind of women of the late 1900s women were made to aspire to, was often white and middle-classed, and therefore of an enviable degree of privilege. The ideal sold to American women, at the time, was of a nature far too limiting to be achievable without sacrifice. Given this fact, consider the weight of the achievements of women like Maya Angelou and Alice Walker, who contributed to our long-standing debate toward equality whilst dealing with systemic racism that was endemic in our society. Remember, even while they were working with a flawed ideology that would ultimately add more burden to their plate, these women took the necessary leap toward making an inconceivable future manifest for the generation that was to follow in their footsteps.

Today's Mom

In light of the past that had women shackled to our households, the 21st century has—to an extent—loosened its leash on women, but at a price. 53% of households today rely on dual incomes (DeMarco, 2021). Surely, this shows that time has established a better means to facilitate equality on both domestic and professional fronts. But what we see is that the cost of living is opening equality while shrinking realistic expectations. The percentage of men who refrained from helping with housework by the early 2000 had fallen to 16%, a steep fall from 30% of husbands completely reported to be uninvolved in 1980 (Hutson, 2018). Husbands have been reported to devote up to 10 hours of their week to housework today which we praise as absolutely incredible— when it happens, although this work is still consistently at least 8 hours behind their wives in doing so. Add that up over a year, and women are spending four-hundred and sixteen additional hours of their time each year doing housework in comparison to the average man. That's the equivalent of 3 weeks vacation to manage one household. In addition to domestic tasks, we can also look at childcare tasks. The amount of time that men spend with their children has tripled since 1965, which does sound fantastic. However, with steps being taken toward making the necessary progress toward social equality, women are simply given the grace to juggle one less ball while still required to handle the arrangements for childcare assistance to take place. Mothers are often the organizers and prepper's for the activities involving their male counterparts, and on many occasions, the clean-up duty for any messes made in the absence of their care. Yes, the modern women of today have the luxury of using advances like washing machines to shorten the hours spent scrubbing their family's clothes, and a comparatively better healthcare system that ensures their protection in childbirth. Though, the disproportionate domestic responsibilities placed on women, mean that they still have much to lose in choosing to become mothers.

The issue with much of our strides toward progress on the prospect of motherhood and the subject of female ambition in the 21st century, is that it merely allow for the ideal of a working woman—leaving much to be desired to actually accommodate her needs comfortably. What America can provide for what some believe to be one of the most hard-working subsections of its population is only a wealth of newer, more difficult decisions. Stay-at-home mothers may be a considerable minority in this brave new world that we embark on together, but this fact doesn't negate how difficult it is to be a mother in the modern era. A figure that encapsulates the lack of support, that stands out starkly in spite of all the changing trends that appear to cater toward our needs, is seven minutes. Between 1997 and 2012, mothers had only enjoyed a relief of a seven-minute decrease in the overall time spent maintaining their households. Boomers may tell you that the wealth of dual-income families exist to make up for the lowered wages of the fathers of our era, but reports show that much of these "two-worker" families are concentrated within higher-income circles that can afford the childcare demanded by the endeavor. Perhaps this is why there exists such a large ideological gap between people on opposite ends of the spectrum. On one hand you have moms from lower-income families, who are forced to become full-time mothers in spite of their other ambitions as a result of a social welfare system that fails to provide for their needs; on the other hand, you have privileged women like Kim Kardashian who believe they have the authority to tell other women to "work" on the flawed belief that they all share the same 24 hours. With the era of the internet, where every opinion is given the opportunity to be placed on a digital pedestal, it doesn't take too much digging to uncover how poorly informed our social stratosphere is on the plight of mothers who do not come from rich, white families.

As a mother who once had to make this decision herself, I can vouch for how emotionally taxing it is to be a stay-at-home mother with no support and no community, when you yearn to contribute to your own mental growth and direct your attention to something fulfilling for your soul rather than repeatedly spending days telling the same stories and counting 1, 2, 3's. Understand that it is not that I didn't enjoy looking after my children, watching them grow, and being their caregiver and influential leader in life. There will never be memories that I cherish as fondly as the bubble baths, silly escapades, and the messy breakfasts I shared with them. Yet, as much as I love my motherhood journey and the whole rat race that comes with it, devoting my entire being to another person didn't turn out to be the best thing I could do for my mental health, and I don't believe it is the best for anyone. In going on autopilot, letting the responsibilities take over my time, I was essentially neglecting my right to my own leisure and wellness. For the first four to five years of my first child's life, my self-esteem was at its lowest. Looking back, it seems strange that I was so oblivious to the impressive amount of vigilance that my mind and body showed in order to make things work. We had just relocated to a little town in Vancouver Island, Canada, for my husband's job. My only support would come from an individual who would be occupied with work during the day— my husband. I found myself nearing my breaking point completely isolated outside of my child as I handled housework and a baby day in and day out for over 3 years. It was kind of like a scene from the show Maid, when the protagonist Alex is subjected to forced isolation from her emotionally abusive parter… only my husband was not abusive, he was just at work for 12 hours and we only had one vehicle which he used to get to work. Childcare was near to nonexistent—and when I did discover some options, I was crushed by how expensive it turned out to be and how long the waiting list was, and how inflexible it was with a shift workers schedule. Moreover, finding a job for me that accommodated the fact that I was a professional who was also a mother— nearly non-existent… shocker.

So, as a large amount of stay-at-home mothers will admit to doing, I blamed myself for the choices that I did not have. I hated that I had to be anchored in my home to keep our family afloat and support my infant all while doing it through a smile to not worry others and make them feel like it was all okay. For some reason, I never thought to blame the circumstances, channeling my dissatisfaction into self-hatred. In my distress, I was blind to how well I was actually doing. Much of the housework and childcare that mothers undertake are often left unthanked. But, in retrospect, as I think of the other factors weighing in on my life, I was only working at the pace that any other mother in my situation would be. Essentially, I simply reflected the narrative that society kept pushing on stay-at-home mothers—that, even in doing it all alone, we are never enough.

Ironically, when I had the opportunity of being in the workforce a couple of years later, society did nothing to accept—never mind celebrate—my accomplishments. Instead of being placed on a pedestal for my efforts, I found myself bombarded by the combined force of my housework and professional duties. Don't get me wrong, my company was accommodating… but only if it didn't effect my job. I was terrified of the unknown happening that would make me look like I wasn't performing. I was constantly worried I would get the call that they were replacing me for someone with no children. Because of this, I worked harder, and stretched myself thinner between my two roles as working professional, and full time mom. In the end, I realized that I had been manipulated into insecurity, shame, and self-hatred because I was backed by a system that—in its promises and bravado—did not want to uphold women. Regardless of your occupation in a potential career or in full-time motherhood, your efforts will likely go unnoticed by the world around you. As exasperating as it must be to read this today, our efforts to raise children are considered to be thankless accomplishments that come with our decision to become a mother. Often, we are denied our due support by people who are far too caught up in their own ways to consider the benefits that institutional change will bring into the lives of women. Mothers of today have to make do with professional lives that do not take into account their motherhood when they exploit their services. Our fine print for ambition includes sick leaves and vacation days spent performing our motherly duties for our kids: tending to functions at their schools, their own bouts of illnesses, birthdays, extracurriculars, and the mountain of other duties that need our active parenting participation. There exists a divide in the realm of parenting, between the reality it prevails to be in the lives of lower-income families and how it is to those privileged enough to shame other mothers who aren't "hustling" as well as they are. Yes, there are more career women than there were 50 years ago. The average age of a first-time mom has risen to 26. Teen pregnancies have decreased significantly. An increased figure of men has been observed to be chipping in on household duties. Yet, this exactly proves where we fall short. Men are still only expected to chip in on their duties toward their families. Households are still pressured to maintain unattainable levels of beauty, and the economic system is built around clocking in workers, instead of supporting wellness and family relationships. The harsh words and ideologies of misogynistic men that caged women in vicious cycles of unpaid labor, have transformed into malignant cultural expectations for things like Instagram worthy homes and full-time boss babes—subjecting women to different breeds of the same toxicity order to attempt thriving in a system not built for them.

Fed Up

I spoke to a mother named Amira. She was a new mom at the age of 23 and she was exhausted. Exhaustion should not be a personality trait. It would probably be more normal for her to introduce herself with her daily occupation or her hobbies; but unfortunately, exhaustion seemed to be a word that is more faithful to her domestic life. Amira is a full-time mother. In this day and age, this is an endeavor that requires you to plate social media-worthy meal plans for your kid—who couldn't care less about what their plate looks like when they mash it, or decide to fling it off their high chair. She struggled to count blessings when things get tough (as they always do, undeniably).

The love that she holds for her one-year-old, in all her bouts of unpredictable rage and random spurts of giggles, is beyond words and time itself. It's just that Amira suffers from one of the most realistic, yet unspoken, difficulties of being a mother. It doesn't take a genius to connect the dots between a baby that has to be trained to sleep through the night to a sleepless caregiver. And yet, there are never words that can define the degree of fatigue that mothers of young children have to grit their teeth through on a daily basis. Repetitive hours of lost rest, is compounding hours of lost recovery and rehabilitation. As an individual without the safety net of a proper support system, it can be incredibly difficult to attempt to preserve energy in a way that prevents burnout when your schedule does not offer you any promises of rest. To the question of when the baby naps, which in and of itself can require much effort to manifest, there's just too much responsibility placed on a mother's shoulders for her to utilize any time for herself. What results are guilty naps that occur like lapses from reality, when the laundry and the pending checklist of to-dos will be spared to give the body a mere trace of the rest that it deserves. She will emotionally pay in guilt later when it's apparent to her husband that she didn't keep the house tidy today. He doesn't have to even say anything, the guilt is just there, and she knows he wonders what she did do all day.

Stories like these are posted almost by the hour on the internet today. Another mother took to ranting on a popular blogging platform to convey her frustrations of being treated less like a person with her own needs because of her motherhood. After nine months of being checked on, regularly and fastidiously, a mother seeking to be looked after post-kids is treated like she is being unreasonable in voicing her needs to those around her. This attitude shown toward mothers who vocally express how difficult parenting is, is cruel in its callousness, but the hurt and rage only worsens when women join in on this behavior, using their privilege as a platform with which they are able to judge women who aren't as lucky as they are. I often wonder how we as women fall into this tigress trap. A friend of mine once said that facing the full force of the responsibilities left for her after the birth of her first child was like waking up to reality, after the illusion of being pampered and doted on for nine months. It probably wouldn't have hurt so much if the pregnancy was treated like the world's most precious miracle. Even if it was, the cold dismissal that comes after the birth of a child feels like being told that all the special treatment had not been for you, but rather solely for the baby inside you. Even as the very backbone that holds her family together, a mother is considered to matter less than her husband and her children in this way. Is this not what the world tells us when it is considered irrational to split chores with a working husband due to our exhaustion? What kind of messages do women receive, when child-centered parenting experts ask them to put their child's feelings first, even when they are yelling and kicking at their mother on the floor of their local grocery store? What are women to do when they are told, repeatedly and consistently, that they will always come second to their families, and no one is coming to their aid?

The moms at Charleston seemed to be having the perfect solution to the problem, choosing to scream out their rage as a form of finding a release. Led by Sarah Harmon, a therapist in their area, a group of moms organized screaming out into the dark streets as a way of venting their frustration at the onset of COVID-19, the lockdown, and the insufferable band-aid online education system with no real support for parents it brought with it. Ironically, these women seemed to have accepted the fact that it was more comforting to roar at empty space than hope for the actual changes that would make things easier for them. The fact that the only relief we have been offered for our struggles as moms is to scream at a literal and disconcerting void makes it evident that we still have much further to go in our journey toward progress. Even when it feels like we have come so far in our struggle to have our rights met and respected, mothers face an ideological divide that makes it impossible for us to pursue normal (if not rested) lives after the birth of our children. If we're ever going to catch a break, It is through structural functionalism where the components of our society—institutions, individuals, culture, traditions, norms, etc.—all work towards a larger goal of caring for the growing human population. It's when we will find ourselves expecting a father to share in *raising* his child, instead of just 'helping out' with childcare for them. It is when a government provides paid support to mothers or caregivers for staying home and raising children. It would be then that we will begin to allow mothers to live their lives as people, and not supermoms, that somehow have the ability to balance the entire world on their shoulders.

Not So Hypothetical: Questions to Ask Yourself

As you reflect on this heavy chapter, take a moment to consider the following questions:

- If you have a partner who you live with, how would you describe the quantity of childcare that they take up when they are at home, and what do weekends look like?
- What rights do you take for granted today that were not readily available to your female ancestors 50 years ago?
- Even if a woman is provided the alternative of a viable career that recognizes her responsibilities to her family, should she be shamed for her decision to become a full-time, stay-at-home mother?
- Is there room in structural functionalism for an admirable duel-working woman and mother, and a fully fulfilled stay-at-home mom?
- Does society have the right to define the terms for an individual's private sense of fulfillment?

- How does privilege—with relation to wealth, race, support, and social status—play into the ease with which women manage motherhood? Can all mothers be attributed the same 24 hours when some have to sacrifice more of their time than others because of a lack of support?
- In what ways do you feel like the world around you has altered its treatment of you after you had children?
- Do you feel like you have been valued less, as an individual, after the birth of your child?

CHAPTER 2

THE INVISIBLE WOMAN

*Through the open door, she sees them all snuggled close
She goes into the room to cover up their little toes.*
—TIARA A. WHITE, "A MOTHER'S STRUGGLE"

Inherent Gender Bias

Saying that you feel invisible as a woman or a mother, in this day and age, will likely earn you several eye-rolls and the title of being the poster child of unachievable feminism. How could you say that women are not being seen, when pushes for equality in the media and various other fields have resulted in feminism being a force to be reckoned with? How dare women have the audacity to make claims about living in a man's world when men have to put up with atrocities like the latest all-female Ghostbusters reboot? —Just kidding on the last one. Regardless of Hollywood's latest gimmicks, female invisibility is a phenomenon that shapes the mobility with which women and mothers navigate the world around them, making them work harder for the same aspects of life that men take for granted. This might seem strange to digest in a world that is hyper-fixated on proving its feminist morale, but facts prove that we evidently inhabit a system that has largely been designed to suit men.

From the gigantic size of current iPhones to the way in which a woman is only guaranteed 30% of her safety in a moving vehicle because leading car companies only thought to use male dummies to simulate accidents, our presence in the world is casually disregarded as if we mattered as much as the male afterthought and did not amount to a good half of the world's population. Caroline Criado Perez, is the writer of the book *Invisible Women*. This book changed my life from the moment I read it. She describes how our day-to-day lives have been designed ideally to suit masculine aspirations, being a struggle against an unseen gender gap. The world is a loud place for opinions right now, and feminist protests and outspoken online presence on feminist rights might seem overwhelming if you have ever dove down the rabbit hole. You may be wondering how such a gender gap is considered to be invisible. The matter with much of our efforts made toward equality is how we simply graze the surface of the issue, instead of digging at its roots as we should be.

Women today are still misdiagnosed for serious health issues because doctors dismiss their symptoms to be imaginary, assuming them to be following the exaggerated behavior that women are believed to epitomize. Doctors' failures to hold statements made by female patients to the same level of faith as a mans words have been dubbed as something called "Yentl Syndrome" and I urge you to look it up— the statistics will shock you! Did you know that the most popular phones on the market were not made for a woman's hand size? They are too large to comfortably hold (thus the cracked screens that we often get and have to pay to fix); female gamers almost always have a hard time balancing gigantic headsets on their skulls; the hand grips on the bus you take home are held on to with ease by the six-foot-tall person that they were designed to accommodate while the average woman stands at 5 foot 4. In 2013, we were made aware of the fact that women take longer than men to metabolize the medication Ambien. The FDA informed us that we are actually supposed to have half the adult dosage of Ambien. Without this vital piece of information, women were taking an excessive amount per dosage, which meant that they would still be under its influence even after several hours of consumption—possibly affecting their reaction time as they drove through busy streets on their way to work or to drop their kids off at school. And, not so surprisingly, according to a 2007 study from the National Sleep Foundation, nearly 3 in 10 American women report using a sleep aid at least a few times a week. This is nearly twice the number of men in the same age group. The conversation statistics show that insomnia in women often starts when they have children. The logistical worries of packing lunches, keeping up with school schedules, and keeping track of everything that needs to be done keeps them awake at night—the invisible work putting the invisible women in harms way.

There have also been findings that if a woman menstruates after taking cardiac drugs prescribed to lessen the risk of a heart attack, she unwittingly achieves the opposite, leaving her life at the brink of stakes that had been raised without her knowledge. Chemicals react differently in the bodies of men and women, even though we are still advised to follow a unilateral adult dosage prescription. Strangely enough, none of the experienced professionals at the pharmaceutical companies that design the drug had considered including menstruating women in their clinical trials which is disturbing considering a study done by the American Heart Association found that Pregnancy-related heart attacks, especially in the period after childbirth, are on the rise in women ages 30 and up. The error could be a fatal one and only adds to the chain of "accidents" that occur because women have been conveniently disregarded as default users for commercial products.

The gender gap plays into elements of our lives as mothers that are as intricate as the routes on a city map. In fact, researchers find that most city maps have been designed to suit the hypothetical nuclear family, that features a working father and a stay-at-home mother (Goode, 2019). The catch in what you would take as a harmless remnant of an outdated world order is that these routes have been designed on the assumption that women would never leave the home, even to pick up a few groceries to cook dinner. These responsibilities would be left to the men, who can leave their work in order to suffice their wives' every need. Only now, women leave the home to shop and their husbands rarely do. Groceries aside, even places like hospitals (which mothers are found to constantly frequent alone in order to care for both their own health and the welfare of their children) have been positioned in places that suit the convenience of working men. The gendered ethics of our world seem to prioritize men above women, working mothers, and especially above stay at home mothers.

So why would something like convenience be such a large issue? Our issue lies in how women have to exert themselves to simply exist in a world that denies its duty to see to their comfort. Women are invisible in this sense. To the figureheads who make the decisions that curate how we are to live our lives, women do not exist. Mothers do not exist; they are the microscopic fine print who risk their lives each time they take their medication when they are on their period; they are the ghosts who constantly reroute themselves through city paths; they are the ethereal bodies who do not drive or play video games, and they are the invisible few who have to accept the fact that they bear 17% of a higher chance of being killed in a car accident (Samuel, 2019).

By this, I do not mean that we are facing a government conspiracy that seeks to protect the ranks of men in society, but that change needs to be recognized in order to create the change that we seek from the world. Criado Perez owes a large portion of the masculine convenience projected to elements of our domestic lives to a gender data gap. As women are left out of the metrics that they should form a vital part of, the products informed by this sexist form of research better fulfill the needs of men than women. It takes a stretch of the imagination for a male, who is a part of a clinical trial procedure, to consider the negative effects that a drug may have on a menstruating woman. Similarly, it is unlikely that male designers and urban planners—or even childless females in these professions—will take the needs of breastfeeding mothers into account as they contemplate the amenities of the latest building or new development layout. One of the most prominent reasons why we feel like we are living in a world crafted for men, by men, is because women and mothers have not been included as spearheads in the important decision-making that impacts our daily lives on this planet.

Recently, Apple blamed Siri's algorithm for the fact that it was reported to be able to look for Viagra but was unable to provide details about abortion clinics. In response to the skeptical eyebrow raised at them, the company has since amended its program's issue of gender bias. Take what you will from that information as it has it's own complexities within it; but similarly many female CVs posted on job sites may not even reach human eyes as they are outright rejected by an algorithm that looks for certain *(hint: male)* features in order to make viable matches to its default high-performing employee template. We can't really blame the software though, can we? After all, a computer knows nothing of prejudice; but this is only the mere surface of the issue that we have to look past. Software can only simulate what it has been taught. Early voice recognition software such as your Alexa or Siri most likely responded to your husband's voice better than your own— Why? It is because it has been fed a greater quantity of male test data. The software recognizes male voices better because it has been made to suit a male default. Trained to respond better to the tenor of a man's voice, the software will inevitably consider female input to be deviations from an established norm. Hence, just as we find ourselves straining to reach the hand grips on public transit on our way to work, we attempt at speaking louder so that our tech can pick up our commands,. We are women repeatedly and unknowingly attempt to compensate for the fact that our domestic products and amenities could use some fine tuning to suit our needs best.

Our invisibility is a phenomenon that we owe to our societal absence backstage, where the ways in which our bodies, lifestyles, and responsibilities distinguish themselves from that of men. We need to be considered valid defaults in all the consideration for products created with the intention of serving the general public. Women—in all our inconvenient differences from pregnancies, to forgotten menstrual cycles, and the need to breastfeed our infants on queue regardless of location in order to keep them alive naturally rather than through formula; have to be considered vital test data. In order to be seen enough for our needs to be met, we should have a stronger presence in the institutions that determine our quality of life.

What happens when these differences bleed into our professional and domestic lives is that we are made to experience a version of the world that is entirely different from that which men do. With the time and effort wasted in making up for the many inconveniences of living in a man's world, we are drained of the energy that could have translated to better job satisfaction, self-esteem, and care for our children with less animosity toward our husbands. Even in fields thought to be relatively neutral in this aspect like academia, which is independent of test data ratios and faulty algorithms, inequality runs rampant in the way in which female professors are provided with lesser work-related opportunities, citations, and salaries than men while they are—at the same time—pressured more for research and job-related endeavors. It shouldn't be surprising to note that women experience less job satisfaction in this field. They are reported to produce fewer overall papers and have smaller collaboration networks than their male counterparts. They are also reported to have spent more time handling childcare responsibilities and household work. Women only make up 32% of our professors; and instead of respecting them for their contributions to their field, they are pushed to their most dire limits almost as if they were compensating for a privilege that would otherwise have been withheld from them (Zheng et al., 2022). Consequently, female professors experience more work-family conflicts than male professors do, despite showing a tendency to have families with fewer children. It would seen that what the statistics suggest is that you have male professors enjoying a work-life balance at leisure while female professors struggle to find a balance between both domestic and work responsibilities that push them to the brink of burnout.

There are some positive moves being made in the right direction however. UN Women seeks to repair the apparent gender bias that causes our chronically prejudiced statistics. Making Every Woman and Girl Count is a program implemented by UN women in order to ensure that women have a significant influence in the way gender-based data are "used, created, and promoted" (Flagship Programme: Making Every, n.d.). And there are a few other notable organizations committed to bringing about a change in gender statistics:

- **The Association for Women's Rights in Development:** Is an organization that advocates for women's rights on the worldwide front. They work to facilitate better dialogue on gender-based discrepancies, aiming to ensure equality in social and financial security that has been granted to women.
- **Gender at Work:** Is an "international feminist knowledge network" aiming to alter the discriminatory practices and cultures embedded within our societies, teaming with researchers and feminist activists in order to pave the way for a more equitable approach to how gender is handled within institutional ethics and internal statistics.
- **Moms Fed Up:** Is an organization devoted to making sure that there are more mothers represented in congress, allowing them to have more control in enacting the legal policies that affect familial needs and wants.

These institutions to build a female presence are a hopeful start to shift our societal gears which mothers need in order to pedal themselves uphill to the summit of change.

Identity Loss

Walking into my first all-moms date felt like taking my first oblivious steps into a war zone. Of course, everyone looked presentable. In the best way that red-eyed mothers can manage their upkeep. I would admire the mom who had taken care to pin her hair back nicely with no flyaways and line her eyes with a little flick that resembled a wing on the edge; we had much in common. We had all woken up early that morning. We all had our preferred caffeine shots at our respective households. Each of us wanted to be a better version of the person seated closest to us I'm sure. Each of us wanted the first impression to be like meeting your friends at the bar in your early 20's— casually strolling in like you didn't put a few solid hours in to look as good as you did. Thinking back to those days when I was living in Ottawa, our polite banters over coffee and mommy workouts seemed pretty irrational. We were all women suffering from the difficulties of parenting in a broken system that went out of its way to make things harder for us. And in this, a good proportion of us (I believe), ran on nonexistent sleep, and we were all under the impression that we were doing less than we should be doing. I got the feeling that we were all hiding our mothering stresses from each other and constantly apologizing with a smile for motherly actions we clearly all related to.

There's a popular cultural belief that parenting should be intensive in nature. Real mothers wouldn't have a hard time trying to care for their vomiting child's gastro issue for the fourth time in the year since they joined preschool. They would just pull up their socks and act on instinct without personally fretting over how gross it was for them. If you were parenting the right way, you would treasure each and every second of it. As an extension of this perspective, there is a view that you should sacrifice not just your individual needs and wants as a person for your children, but pretend that they don't exist at all. Even without realizing it myself, reading about intensive parenting showed me how the toxic positivity had begun to get to me. I wanted my child to have the best possible life that I could grant him. Obsessed with this want, I told myself that all I had to do was let my body survive. I was fine living on survival mode for years before I could consider prioritizing myself over my little human again. Intensive parenting has been linked to a plethora of mental illness issues that emphasize how it may probably not be the best parenting methodology out there. I hadn't known this when I forced myself to wait (sometimes an hour or two) till the baby slept so I could use the bathroom. I hadn't known this, on the days when I tried to convince myself that a full-time job would pull away my children's opportunities to thrive, telling myself it was my duty to stay home with them and be fully present day and night until at least the age of five. With my two kids, three years apart... that is eight years of feeling invested in a delusion.

Research has shown us how incredibly difficult it is for mothers to exist while centering their lives around their babies; reportedly connecting this approach to a higher risk of falling into depressive disorders. This should not be surprising. After all, we shouldn't expect people to be able to cope well with a sudden loss of identity and purpose. This is not to say that you cannot find purpose in your child, but doing so in a way that leaves you tending to their needs above your own can perpetuate an unhealthy relationship between the both of you. When I told myself that I would make up for the loss of my job by becoming the best mother I could be for my child, I found myself worn out by how I was unable to find satisfaction in their carefully structured meal plans and routine activities on the days they were fussy. On the many occasions that I lost my cool when my children cried, peed their pants, or broke an important family heirloom that has been hanging on the wall (yes this happened); I berated myself for not mothering well enough to enjoy every second of the time I spent with them. Heedless of the fact that I had a right to my own feelings—just as my children had a right to their tantrums and desire to stray from the little bubble of perfection that I had placed them in—I pushed myself to be pleased with a life that constantly demanded my resourceful patience. This left me ultimately and inevitably falling into the pit of burnout that would leave my mind in an utter mess for weeks looking for anxiety relief in CBD oils, breath techniques, and attempted audio guided meditation sometimes with tears running down my face while I picked up the kids toys and cooked dinner before my husband came home.

This is why it is so important that women are supported in their desire to find occupations or purpose outside of their motherhood. The system that is currently in place for us expects mothers to be okay with losing their career-related aspirations and pre-kid identity to the exciting life of mothering alone; a life that demands women to remain on their feet for the entirety of their days (and not requiring to be praised or simply thanked for their efforts); a life where mothers who wish to seek career opportunities to meet the demands of acquiring a semblance of stability, means that she often has to live without her mother, or other related family, at hand to support her in raising children. We have come to be so divided in our hunt for economic stability. Our system denies mothers affordable childcare, flexible work hours, and domestic help, leaving no alternative for a life that is isolating in how it revolves around the sacrificial caretaking of young children. If you have spent time alone, in isolation with your child for extended periods of time, and you have felt this way— it is no fault of your own. Men, traditionally, have little to no obstacles placed in the way that disallows them from enjoying their families as well as their work.

In spite of our supposed progress, society still expects women to handle housework and childcare by themselves. Mothers currently wage through a gender gap forced by both ideological and institutional fronts. As I mentioned earlier, even when mothers are in positions of prominence in the workforce, our deeply flawed conception of gender roles results in mothers chewing off more than they can swallow. After becoming a father, one of my husband's morning tasks on weekends involved getting up and making himself coffee, and sitting down to a video game for a few hours. The same was for when he returned home from work during the week. After all, a hard day at work deserves a much needed break. He would shower and pick out his clothes and always look nice. Studies show that becoming uncaring of your appearance was one of the red flags of depressive disorders, and I suppose my husband was looking out for himself in opting for coordinated outfits when he was not at work. Still, I remember my resentment for his rather nice appearance that made me attracted to him. I hated how put-together he was when mothering left me no time to have a skincare routine, style my crazy wavy hair, shave, or be inclined to wear something other than sweatpants and the same shirt I took off before my three-minute shower if I was lucky; I knew my husband hated that shirt too. Caring for my toddler around the clock meant that I barely had time to work out or indulge in any of the self-care activities that all those rich Instagram moms always raved about. Motherhood changed the way I looked and changed the way I saw myself. I was always dirtier than I wanted to be. There was always something about myself that I wanted to straighten up but didn't have the time or the patience to do so. With time, I grew numb to the specifics and tried to convince myself that I didn't care. There were just so many invisible tasks that were automatically assumed to be my responsibility, that the upkeep and maintenance of my appearance grew to become a *want* that I did not have the luxury of fulfilling. Instead, I kept my hair in its messy bun and tended to the laundry that I was always a few days behind on.

A highly qualified woman—I will call her "Jane" backed by a prestigious degree and master's certificates described to me one of her many losses in the journey of motherhood to be her desk job. After four kids, Jane faced a huge lapse in finding a sustainable career path. Years of being off the horse had left her a mountain of pending work that she had yet to catch up on. Family-friendly jobs were less of a rarity than they had been when she had first left her job in order to look after her first child, but finding a job that suited her expertise with a payout that made it worth the expenses in childcare was like finding a needle in a haystack. Even when it was made apparent to her that she had a high chance of being successfully recruited back into the workforce, the logistics of parenting are such that time is often made too unpredictable to be molded to suit the framework of a second occupation with unpredictable hours and related commitments. If she dove back into the job force, her husband would have to make sacrifices. She felt guilty to even bring up the conversation with him. What results is a highly qualified professional, who has been given no alternative but to place her education and her achievements on the back burner, struggling with the concept of being forced to identify with a version of their own life that they cannot relate with. Any women like Jane, should not have to choose between having children and having a career. Becoming a mother should not have to translate to an inevitable loss of purpose and identity. While it may be easy for us to attribute the obvious joy that children bring to compensate for the drastic loss of identity that women have to contend with, such a line of thought conveniently compels women to make choices that make up for the plethora of work left to be fulfilled by the world around them.

The workforce, even when it no longer banned pregnant women from their office desks, still had a long way to go in ensuring equality in the way that it meets the needs of all its employees. Forty-three percent of highly qualified professionals are reported to be leaving work, both permanently and for temporary periods of time (Light, 2013). The effort that has been put into supporting mothers at work currently falls short of what they require in order to have a work-life balance that is free of stress. Our service to the workforce should not be treated as a privilege, as if we were simply inexperienced children who should be grateful to have been given a chance to earn money in spite of our own shortcomings. The labor required from a working mother causes her to essentially slave away at both her home and her workplace in order to meet the unreasonable expectations placed on her. As a mother who struggles to manage a 40-hour work-from-home schedule single-handedly, I find that I can very much resonate with the feeling that our system scams us of our services without making its own contributions, which have long been overdue.

The most frustrating part about the gap between the work-life balance experienced by professionals who are mothers and those who are fathers is that it is not a situation beyond repair. Although it may take a lot of effort to bring things to a level where men and women can have an equitable life experience, an awareness of the gender gap and the way in which women can bridge their way across it may allow for changes that lessen the burden placed on women to a significant extent.

Conscious alterations made to the domestic and workplace norms that could help lessen the load for working moms should include:

- the presentation of close-end projects, with clear time frames set for client objectives, allowing parents to have foresight in scheduling their work week around their family commitments
- splitting unpaid domestic labor more equitably with a partner, if they are present
- making affordable childcare a reality
- changing public transit routes in a way that accommodates the day-to-day travel needs of working women
- including diverse groups of women in trials for commercial products
- pushing for more political visibility for women, especially mothers, so that public spaces accommodate their needs

- allowing mothers the leeway that they deserve, given the overwhelming degree of responsibilities placed on their shoulders

What we as a society need to provide for the mothers of our populations is validation and support. Mothers are reported to be sleep-deprived for the first 6 years of their children's lives. Unlike the popular belief that concentrates sleep deprivation and other childcare-related difficulties as issues that only occur in the first two years of life, studies have proven that what parents do sacrifice are years' worth of their health to tend to their children. The modern woman is facing a struggle to manage her career and her household in a gender gap that is both ideological and institutional.

If you find yourself disheartened by the giants that stand before your visibility in the world, and the struggle that awaits you in the years to come. For now, hold on tight. Do the best that you can do, and in a way that doesn't drain you of your energy. If that means you will be letting your toddler walk around in juice stained clothes in a while instead of waging war with him over changing into a clean shirt as you often find yourself doing, know that you are doing fine—if not perfect. Motherhood should never be about accuracy. It should never be about ticking someone's invisible checklist or coordinating earth tones in their outfits when they want to wear a princess dress, because these things truly do not matter. Think of it this way: Whichever way you put it, mothering is hard. It was hard in the 19th century when the men handled the schoolwork, it is hard now when your children actually do their homework under the supervision of an online tutor even. It is hard when you don't get a good night sleep because all they want to do is cuddle you, and you know these will always be the precious moments. Being a mother is difficult. It leaves too much to assume and has the quality of triggering men (and despairingly more-so sexist men). Working nine-to-five jobs is a another story entirely, with awful management systems that leave you worn to the bone by the time you finally get to leave work. Needless to say, it would be impossible to be all three of these demanding roles (mother, educator, and worker) together. Even if that little voice in your head attempts to convince you about how amazing *super-momming* would be, remind yourself that the loss of sleep and mental stress is not worth it. Instead, train yourself to view your parenting and work duties to be second to your sense of comfort as long as safety is covered. If you feel too tired to bake your kids cookies from scratch after a long day of work, opt for a prepackaged snack. If your laundry induces most of the anxiety that you have in relation to maintaining your home, move this responsibility to your partner's daily list of to-dos instead of your own, or create a system of practise for the family that allows you a break if your children are old enough. A chore basket with laminate chore cards is a great way to implement this. Kids can pick a chore card from the basket, complete the task, and trade that chore card in for a reward like screen time. Although you may find yourself yearning for an all-encompassing wave of change that will transform the way that you lead your life, you must recognize the benefits of the baby steps.

To achieve the collateral change that you desire, you may benefit by adopting some of these approaches:

- Let go of the little habits that you picked up on the way to becoming an ideal of a perfect working mother. That means letting go of holding yourself to the expectation of super-mom, ready to pick up and be the default parent, or plan the month out for the entire family.
- Let go of the need to prove to anyone, be it your boss or your partner, that you are the perfect parent. Perfection does not exist. We need to break the stigma of expressing the difficulties of mothering when our domestic efforts have been popularly

thought of as one of the many invisible responsibilities of motherhood.

- Accept that you may not always be in control of your life, or that of your child. An unhealthy habit that many mothers fall prey to is helicopter parenting—or attempting to control every minute aspect of their children's lives—in order to create a semblance of authority that they can reassure themselves with. Motherhood will always be unpredictable. You cannot change this, because your child has a right to their spontaneity. You can cope with the prospect of never knowing what your day may be like by learning to embrace unpredictability instead of berating yourself for failing the impossible task of controlling the situation— Trust yourself to let go a little.
- Grant new mothers the emotional support they need. If you can, be that help to allow a friend due time to rest and recharge, or encourage other people to volunteer and look after the baby for a while or help out with the housework. We all need to support each other even if you have not granted the same luxuries—pay it forward.
- Help to make financial support more readily available to new parents who may be struggling financially by advocating for it. Research observing the way families who were eligible for the Earned Income Tax Credit fared in parenting in comparison to those that were not, showed that financial support and tax breaks during the early years of parenting can have a significant effect on the education and development of the children concerned. Think of how much a cash investment would have helped you at a time when you had been struggling to make ends meet. Not only could it have given you the security that you needed at the time, but it would have also ensured that you were in a better mental space. Low-income families cannot provide the same opportunities to their children that are made exclusive

by economic differences. Advocating for change in financial support to lower income families could make a generational difference.

- Normalize speaking about your family and family commitments in the workplace, and vice versa. Neither of your roles at the office or your home has to be exclusive of each other. You do not have to work like you do not have the responsibility of raising children, and you do not have to raise children in a way that does not acknowledge your work commitments. The working mother should be recognized as a role in its own right. Refraining from coupling the two will only leave you to juggle roles that do not allow room for each other. If you are comfortable with it, express your feelings to those around you. There could be occasions when your bravery will result in allowing yourself, and other mother's relief, as a vouch for the invisible struggles. You may be surprised at the type of movement and change that you can start.
- Realize that a large part of your struggles come from an institutionalized gender gap. Even if you feel like you have heard these words enough times to remove the gist of their meaning, *it's not your fault*. You are fighting against a broken system that fails to recognize women and mothers. The sooner you let yourself recognize the consequences of this fact, the sooner you will let go of the practice of chasing unattainable perfection. For this reason alone, even when you feel like you're doing your worst—you are truly doing great.

Not So Hypothetical: Questions to Ask Yourself

Reflect on the following questions, and write your answers down if you wish:

- In what ways has the gender data gap affected you negatively? Have you ever been misdiagnosed, or treated differently in a medical context because you are a woman?
- In what ways do you believe our world is crafted for men by men? Has there been a change in this trend? If so, how?
- How does the gender gap play into motherhood for you and the choice that women often have to make between their families and their careers?
- What are the ways in which you feel invisible as a woman to the world around you?
- How do you think the gender gap could be bridged?

CHAPTER 3

THE DEFAULT PARENT

> "The thing about parenting rules is there aren't any. That's what makes it so difficult."
> —EWAN MCGREGOR

Upon accepting her award for Best Actress in a Motion Picture—Drama, Glenn Close was moved to tears by the honor the prestigious title granted her, as one might expect her to be. There was one particular aspect of her speech though, that struck a strong chord with the audience and it's viewers. The highlight of Close's speech ended up being her mother, who–at the age of 80—was quoted to have said, "I feel like I haven't accomplished anything" (Kosin, 2019). The statement drew a powerful reminder of how easily women can lose their individuality in their pursuit of providing for their families. In spite of how wealthy and famous an individual Glenn Close was, and how massively successful *The Wife* (a movie clustered with several themes of womanhood, marriage, and femininity) had become, there was something about her mother's words that so many people found achingly familiar. Surprisingly, the discourse that the statement had stirred up hadn't only been limited to 80-year-olds who felt like their existence lacked fulfillment. Women of a diverse range of ages, races, and cultures resonated with the quintessential feeling, which could perhaps be more acutely defined as a fear of being oblivious to your own loss of purpose.

The reality of womanhood, and the choices that we are inclined to take, is that much of our energy is often spent looking after other people. While the image of an existence of 80 years accounting for nothing more than servitude to a husband, or a family, may appear horrendous to some, research shows that we aren't high up enough in our ladders to personal success that we can dismiss this fear. If not for feeling like we have accomplished nothing, we feel like we have lost purpose in our accomplishments—as if the strain of pushing ourselves in-between work and home will wear us thin. The prospect of so much effort ultimately resulting in meaninglessness is chilling in the implications that it holds for women, who are at crossroads about the decisions they have to make regarding their career, their families, and their life.

Close describes her mother to have occupied herself for a span of a lifetime in "nurturing" her husband and children. With our system providing such a poor level of support for working women and exerting such a ghastly amount of pressure on stay-at-home mothers to conform to its unattainable standards, women are constantly pushed toward taking the role of nurturing their loved ones. Having someone in your family whom you can always turn to for support may seem like a comforting idea, on paper—but this conventional ideal of a mother being the default caretaker of a household comes with its own repercussions. Of course, it is convenient when women are content with being the caretaker, the nurturer, and the housekeeper. You don't need to look too far when you want answers to all your problems and life tends to have a quality of smoothness when its entire upkeep is delegated to a single individual. However, this role—in all its glory—is also exhausting and extremely lonely. In the networked, massive families of our past—where aunts, uncles, and grandparents lived under the same roof— the workload may not have been so heavy. Sometimes, the issue is not about the weight at all, but about how it is considered fair to limit one person when the other is allowed absolute liberty in their personal, professional, and domestic lives. There is a depth of privacy that my husband enjoys in comparison to myself, who has had to share my workspace, self-care time, meals, showers, and naps with my children by default. There may be an ease with which a woman may be considered the default parent, but this sense of convenience does not come close to equalizing the loss of freedom and individuality that women often owe to this role without question.

In looking after other people, women sacrifice their time and—too often—their health in order to constantly be of service. Much of the work that women do on a daily basis can be translated into unpaid domestic labor. Housework, cooking, and childcare—tasks that may be rendered trivial in comparison to an office job, but amount to their own sense of value if done through hired help—often fall to the hands of the women of the family. Strangely enough, even when these tasks are attributed to hired help, they are dominated by the female sex. Our babysitters, elementary and kindergarten teachers, midwives, and housekeepers are rarely ever men. It's almost as if it is beneath masculinity to contribute to the tasks that men have defined as a woman's job. The split in gender roles may have made sense when men were out hunting, but in todays world, men are not exerting themselves through what we consider masculine traits. Instead, fathers are out for the day, perhaps sitting in an office chair socializing with other male workers and younger female counterparts. It feeds a new kind of masculinity that feels as if it is intended to divide a healthy family bond. It weakens the relationships between not only husbands and wives, but also fathers and their children. Even as these things are slowly beginning to change, they are hardly changing at a pace that women from minority, low-income households can imagine benefitting from in the near future. Think of your own community and the elders that its values are surely rooted in. Think of your friends and colleagues who are not too invested in the many issues that relate to inequality; would they be accepting of a househusband, who would find themselves concerned with housework and childcare, being entirely dependent on his breadwinner wife the same way that they would accept a housewife of similar qualities? It's extremely difficult to imagine, isn't it? The silent qualities that *good* women are often esteemed for possessing would not amount to the same value for men, nor can we believe men would accept such a stark inequality even if it meant his wife and children's comfort was secured by his painstaking devotion to his househusband role. Hypothetical role reversal often reveals privileged ignorance.

If you feel like we're reading too deeply into things that are already considered to be an intrinsic part of our society because many women enjoy cooking and most women don't mind housework as well, you would feel women are naturally inclined to be empathetic toward others. It fortifies why women are society's best caretakers! Obviously, every mother loves her child more than life itself! Labeling childcare as labor would probably even seem appalling to some. These sentiments are true, but they miss the mark in quantifying domestic efforts. What is often left out of the equation is the dismissal of the education of the women through career growth, and also the blatant assumption that their time is less valuable than that of their male counterparts.

Think about this: Even for work that has to be paid for in her absence, a woman's work is insistently considered to be an inherent part of her nature. Women are expected not to mind spending the time that they could otherwise balance more fruitfully to tend to important personal needs. This could be in terms of her mental health and also with relation to monetary means, in the light of the greater good that is taking care of their family. Perhaps, a woman's needs are conveniently considered to possess less value than that of the others in her family, thankfully being limited to the satisfaction that she undoubtedly gains in pleasing others. Maybe it is just easier to imagine that a woman has no needs outside the need to fulfill the work that has to be done in order to make sure everyone has a smooth day. When someone falls sick, wants food on their table, has their babysitter bail on them, or simply needs someone to lean on, you can always count on the women of the house to be of service. Who, then, looks after the mother? Who are their natural caretakers? Part of a mothers mythical qualities is self-sufficiency. Mothers, grandmothers, aunts, sisters, and other females may help bring up a little girl—but when she grows up, there will be no one left to tend to her as she would be committed to nurturing a family of her own. Never mind that a woman is an individual too, equipped with her own emotional needs often left ignored. Our system places so much on her plate that a woman is outside the range of the basic demands of existence, being too busy with her chores to have time for anything else. Older sisters often take on responsibilities as young as ten years old, becoming the secondary default caregiver to the mother instead of the father, and even more so if a mother is a single caregiver of multiple children.

A mothers payless full work day is accomplished silently and without acknowledgment. It's engrained on our daughters from a young age. You see, thanking someone who sets the table, changes the sheets, and washes dirty laundry on the daily, runs the risk of letting them know the value of this work, which goes against what the system wants us to believe. Let them think it is easy. If they don't believe you, try convincing them that they aren't doing anything special. What a patriarchal society achieves when it simply expects women to be tireless workers of its broken system, is deceiving them about the nature of the lives they live. Mothers are fed many lies. We are told that we must conform to the cultural norms around us, even when they stifle our innermost sense of creativity. We are told that we must accept the fact that we are to live within reach of our desires, caged in a way that we can only feel a trace of our true potential. Again and again, we are fed the lie that we must sacrifice our lives for our children rather than grow with them. The narrative that we find ourselves eclipsed in subjects children to be the unwitting catch-22s of our lives. The patriarchy will tell us to blame our children, who are incapable of complex speech and rely on us to thrive. Our system markets childbirth to be a fulfilling act, and only secretly exhausting, incredibly painful and life threatening. Resentment is not a closeted feeling that women wish to hold within themselves, nor should they have to even consider it if we were to be valued in our own respective feminine way. Don't let them gaslight your feelings, because as powerful as our emotions may be, they can only begin to take their footpath toward change by being spoken out loud. The silence that we are encouraged to uphold is a subtle fix that perpetuates the cycle of repression women find themselves in.

Once again, a difference of opinion may surface here, as you think women have achieved too much in western society to still be considered victims of the patriarchy. What most people overlook is that the feminist revolution, in all the milestones that it was able to bring us, had limits of its own and a political agenda. Without the momentous changes brought about in the past decade, single white women may not find it as easy as they do today to have a life centered on a career without constraints pushing them toward marriage and children. However, the same ease with which this group commands their professional lives cannot be attributed to women of various other races, cultures, and identities. Our broken system fails to accommodate women with children, and women of color, in the same way that it tends to single white women. It is Ironic that the ease with which some men and women are able to maintain a successful balance between their professional and domestic lives is owed only to the efforts of other women, who are underpaid for the housework and childcare duties that they perform for the household. A woman from a low-income background, stepping in to fill the gap. A woman who faces the prospect of a potential pregnancy herself, and still has to consider having to sacrifice her job and future career aspirations. The change that we need, in order to allow women to enjoy the same liberty with their domestic and professional lives that men take for granted, has to be brought about by a grassroots movement. Women have reached the limits of the progress they are able to enact. There needs to be men who are willing to step up for change. There exists toxic cultural ideologies that have to be broken down. What stands before us is a task that society needs to be made accountable for. Women have done their part. Is it possible to direct responsibility where it is truly due? It is time for husbands to stand with their wives.

How Women Became the Default Parent

When a child is first conceived, their mother is placed on a pedestal for achieving conception. Miraculously, as evidence of the undeniable force of human nature that repeats itself like a timeless melody, a pregnancy has occurred. New life has been created within a single body. The physicality and emotional weight of this fact alone, accompanied by other—and less reputable—realities that come with it, make the mother and the child a unit of their bond. Bound by fate, and an umbilical cord that turns a woman into both a manifestation of majesty and also a nauseous, awkward mess, the baby and the mother begin their journey together. This strange combination, of mythical greatness and practical inconvenience, continues for a period of nine months—until that final baited cry of life, when birth occurs. This may seem like a rather accelerated and somewhat sarcastic look at how baby and mother bond, but the act of becoming a mother is in itself the single most virtuously diminished miracle we as humans can experience. Of course, birth only heightens the monumental nature of a mother's existence to serve. A baby has to be fed by the breast, which inevitably belongs to its mother. A baby has to be bathed, changed, understood—more than not by the mother who takes on these responsibilities more naturally by default in the first days, all while her aching body is downplayed for the care that it deserves to be showered with. The care pattern continues well after the baby is weaned and introduced to formula milk or solid foods out of sheer routine. When a baby speaks it's first words and and when a child

THE DEFAULT PARENT

can stand on their own, it is the mother who inevitably continues these progressive parenting duties. Eventually, it is agreed—without words and fanfare—that it is the mother who will frequent school meetings, recitals, sports meets, and doctor's appointments. She *is* the mother, after all. Shouldn't she care to tend to her child's every need as it has evolved that way from birth without question?

I spoke to a friend Emma who ended up becoming the default parent because her husband Jacob was too busy to do so. His job demanded that he would be at his office pretty much from 7 a.m. to 7 p.m. It was obvious he wouldn't be able to expend his work hours for the care of the child that he was working so hard to support. She understood that he would be too tired when he showed up at home after taking the late-night commute, and maybe throwing in a few post-work drinks with his colleagues to tend to an irritable baby once or twice a week. Jacob loves his baby; his little girl is the love of his life—just like his wife, who gave up a career as a marketing executive to be a stay-at-home (default) parent. It is just when Emma gets cranky about having a life of her own, that he feels tested. A long day is a tiring endeavor. Emma should know better right? He works hard to support his family and misses his girls, and he learned from his mother that being a mum is all about sacrifices. By paying the bills that provide for the household, he partakes in the duty of supporting. Emma does not earn money, so she should be content with being a stay-at-home mother. Only, she finds that her new occupation has left her more exhausted than her previous nine-to-five, which isn't too surprising. Her days are successions of little struggles.

Her baby has to be fed, cleaned, and entertained before he feels like he can sleep. His nap period is a short lapse of time that took a lot of training to master him into accepting. She feels this nap time can be an opportunity to do something for herself, but God only knows how long his nap will truly last— I can relate to this one. Emma does the groceries, cleans, and cooks lunch before her baby's grand awakening, and the cycle repeats. Emma has no work-free Sundays. She doesn't see the point of taking a day off cleaning if it only means that she would have more work to do on Monday. On a daily basis, she has her exhaustion to battle with. If a little sleep is missed the night before, it compounds throughout the week. Emma has no vacation days to look forward to. On the occasion that she wants to go outside and socialize with her friends, her husband fails to really understand how important this is to her and makes her feel like she is taking time away from the family when he is home. He also needs his rest on his Sundays, even when she only wishes for a few hours. He asks her if she could ask her mother, her sister, or a babysitter to watch the little one on these days. Sometimes, he suggests that she take their baby with her. Her friends probably wouldn't mind. The issue is, it hurts Emma deeply to see him so turned off by the work that she never bats an eye at. It's so easy for him to make alternative suggestions, but never take her up on balancing the load. He never seems to understand that she is an individual in her own right, that she needs some time on her own—free of the backdrop of tending to her child. There lies a clear divide between her life before and after she had children. Emma can't help but miss the person she used to be, who—for one—had the privilege of having an equitable relationship with her husband. What is important to note about Emma's situation is that her husband is not in any way a bad husband or father; he was simply raised to believe that his wife would take on the same role as his mother did, regardless of how the world around them had changed in the last few decades.

Zoe is another mother I spoke to. In Zoe's case, she had been a lawyer before she had been a mother. After making the decision to leave her practice to tend to her children, Zoe took on the role of a stay-at-home mom for six long, beautiful, messy years. Presently, she has two children, who are both in school. As she watched her second child make his first steps into preschool, leaving her mornings irresistibly free, she felt a deep sense of ache settle in her chest. Zoe loves her kids. They come first to her, before her husband, her career, and certainly before herself. Still, she couldn't help but feel like all her experience and intellectual capacities were being put to waste in the archives of her dusty unused portions of her mind. Zoe could handle pages upon pages of someone's messy legal profile, and her most important concerns seemed to lie in things like picking the best laundry detergent to avoid an itchy rash on sensitive skin while still getting out grass stains. Back when they were little, and they had been dependent on her for basic survival needs—Zoe had found fulfillment in the way her family needed her. Now that her children were older, and beginning to grow independent, she knew that she needed to make her own brave steps into the world again where others would recognize her as more than a mother.

She picked morning classes at a local university. Her class only met up three times a week, so she would still manage to be home before the kids came back from school. A little bit of meal prep and some takeout meant that Zoe could make a tentative start to a new career. However, as good things are often coupled with, fate brought the unexpected cold and flu cycle in with the change of seasons. Every other week, someone in her kids' classes would catch a virus of some sort, and they would have to stay home. It was post pandemic, so there was no other choice. Her morning classes were hit the hardest by the change in plans. It wasn't like her husband couldn't pitch in, but he wouldn't unless she nagged, and that something Zoe didn't want to do. Her classes only took a couple of hours, at most; she wished he would offer to help. He managed a business that allowed him to set his schedule how he needed with quite a bit of flexibility, but he chose to take long lunches in the office on days he could spare the time at home to help out. It was easier not to commute back and forth, and it felt good to be back in the office after Covid. So whenever it came to the kids, Zoe had to be the one who did the heavy lifting. They were her responsibility, even when he could help her tend to them. He helped out fairly enough, but going out of his way to support her seemed to be out of the question. It wasn't even intentional. He simply didn't understand his privilege. She had to make her sacrifices. It was like her aspirations were something that only non existent time would permit her to do, as if his convenience formed the jurisdiction for Zoe's life. She was the woman, after all, like Cinderella that had too many household duties (from society) preventing her from going to the ball.

What these mothers share in common is:

- a guilty conscience that makes them feel solely responsible for their children
- the unfair burden of being the default parent
- partners who fail to understand their need to have their aspirations exclusive of parenting their children
- partners that are not considered, or do not want to be considered, as the default parent
- hectic lives
- messy schedules
- exhaustion

It is unsurprising that women fall prey to a toxic form of servitude to their families. This may sound a bit too harsh, but I believe that a willingness to be honest about the issues that we face as men and women would help us lower our pointed fingers and work on the fundamental changes that we have to enact (in both our domestic and professional spaces) if we are to reach equality. In most contexts, a mother's career is almost unquestionably considered to be beneath her maternity. Leaving this belief to your subjective opinion, I believe that most women may be able to agree that the work undertaken by both parents should be considered equitable for a more progressive future. If both parents are able to leave work, how come it is often the woman who is considered to be more likely to take up childcare when the situation demands it? As a society, why is the mother often the first to be called when there is an issue concerning her child? As we watch women drop off kids at school, pick them up for doctor's appointments, take them to extracurriculars, and leave work to tend to them—a father's level of detachment from his children only grows increasingly apparent. With more women driving, taking up jobs, and also handling the household chores typically attributed to men in the past, a father's role in this continues to diminish in size and prominence. We need to think about cultural trends and assess how they shape our lives, instead of passing them to future generations like a pair of outsized shackles. We need to consider in retrospect the problematic nature of our practices. The change will be awkward at first. Sometimes, the decisions that you will have to make may seem strange against the backdrop of the decisions made by the older generations of women in your family. Do not let yourself be limited by this. Modern mothering should break the chain of conformity that hung heavy in the lives of women before us—if not for ourselves, but for our daughters, and the sons who need to be taught to respect and support the women and mothers around them. As we consider the task before us, we may be overwhelmed by its volume, growing insecure about our own abilities to fight it. Remember that we cannot help facilitate a system that dismisses women—and women's rights—entirely. We so easily give in; we so easily help others before ourselves. Even if it seems impossible today, it is the bravery of the women who stood behind us, in the last century, that has accounted for the comparative ease with which we live our lives today. I challenge you to carry this bravery in your heart and allow it to be your source of strength. If anyone can do it, it is you, Mama—you have held the weight of the world on your capable shoulders more than once already. Questioning which traditions serve both men, women, and children for the better, and discarding anything that no longer serves desired modern family structures, is the first step to reconstructing nuclear family roles and values which are established upon the tasks shared within the home.

Not So Hypothetical: Questions to Ask Yourself

As you have reached the end of this chapter, I want you to consider the following questions:

- Are dissatisfaction and purposelessness about oneself, feelings that are commonly felt by any mothers you know? Are they felt by you?
- In what ways do you conform to the notion that insists on women's natural ability to nurture those around them and not just their children?
- Growing up, women are looked after by the women around them. Their mothers, grandmothers, aunts, and sisters frequently ensure that their needs are being met. However, as they grow up, choose partners, and have families of their own, they are often considered to be nurturers without anyone left to look after their own emotional needs. Can you relate to this pattern? Does it contribute to your sense of loss?
- In what ways would you consider the emphasis that is often placed on the mother-child bond to be isolating? In what ways had your experiences with parenting in the early days of your infant's life empowered, or negatively impacted, your identity as a woman?

CHAPTER 4

THE PRESSURES OF MOTHERHOOD

"How wild it was, to let it be."
—CHERYL STRAYED

The Myth of Motherhood

Cassandra is a mommy blogger. If you are familiar with this particular variant of social media influencing, it involves aesthetically pleasing rooms and plating arrangements that toddler eyes, in all honesty, do not even care about. Her Instagram is a picturesque vision of what motherhood ought to be like. Beautiful, urine free sheets that go well against the room's thematic dusty beige. Even her daughter—the daughter who is only pictured donning meticulous French braids—seems to edge on Cassandra's level of perfection. Of course her daughter has the days where she throws the laundry down their Spanish balcony. However, she is potty-trained and knows how to feed herself at the meager age of two and a half. Cassandra makes sure to include disclaimers that assure viewers of the actual behind-the-scenes of her haven of a home. Still, she always gets asked how she manages to "do it all."

To most of her viewers, Cassandra is perfect in all the ways that count. She runs a business of her own, selling perfumes and pastel-colored baby clothes that put most adult clothes to shame in their own brand of self-contained modesty. She makes her meals by herself. To all eyes, she is a supermom. However, as Cassandra reads message upon message sent by desperate mothers seeking to attain her level of perfection, she feels like a liar. She never intended to imply that she did it all. She hadn't known that she was expected to do so at the start, but she still molded into the lie of expectation she was held to. Her successful mothering is supported by her mother (who lives next door to her) and by her husband, who is a work-from-home business manager for their growing family brand. Cassandra drops her kids off at her mother's place in the evenings, when she needs a bit of time to edit the next video post, manage invoicing—or sit and simply sleep if she needs. She orders takeout when she doesn't feel like cooking. Her husband makes a point of taking their family out on Fridays and cooking dinner three times a week. Cassandra's emotional support system is cemented by the days she pretends she doesn't have to juggle her work with the responsibilities that she owes to her children. No one on the gram sees this.

Filled with guilt, Cassandra comes clean. She informs her audience of her support system and the transformative effect that it can have on raising young children. She supposes that this will help normalize the division of labor in households with children. To her surprise, her confessions are met with negativity. How *dare* she have the audacity to gloat about her luck? How could she burden her loved ones with her children's demands when she was there to do it? Her husband needed his energy. Her mother deserved rest in her seniority. As a grown woman, Cassandra should be able to manage her household by herself, if she wanted to be respected. This can all be done even in the perfect life pin-holed through an iPhone camera— Right?

The existence of a supermom has preceded our generation. Before the high-resolution photographs of perfectly dressed young women coddling multiple children, came the mother who showed up to parties with her consciously mannered angels in tow. She is the mother on the bus, who lugs a cello for her daughter on their way to practice recitals. She is the mother who always had a home-cooked meal, packed neatly in her child's lunch box, along with fruit and cookies made from scratch the night before. If you look hard enough, you will find her all around you. It is not difficult to be hyperconscious of insecurities and let yourself become consumed by the self-hatred that society pushes women into falling prey to. It is easy to look at another woman and envy how she seems to be doing a better job at maintaining her household than you are. It is even easier to berate other women, who aren't struggling as hard as you are to uphold the regressive expectations that you strive to maintain. We all want to maintain flourishing careers, beautiful homes, and healthy meal plans to a level of absolute excellence, but consider that maybe all of this toxicity around *doing it* only exists because it is so hard to do so. The issue with the benchmark that mothers are given, is that it is an unreliable measure of her true performance. Sit and let that stew for a moment… Even when you excel at your work goals or presentation and you meet 'the bar', society will always find some facet of your character that fails to meet their expectations for you and the bar will raise. Oftentimes when this happens, we will sit back and suck up the toxic kool-aid to spit in each others faces because social media has created the perfect breeding ground for it. This height of chasing perfectionism is alarmingly displayed in a 2016 episode of Black Mirror titled *Nosedive*. The main character Lacie hits rock bottom in the pursuit of social acceptance she believes will bring her happiness and fulfilment in a paradoxal matrix of her modern society that she is simply living in to follow; though in this paradigm… she is childless. The concept of self implosion through the hunt for perfection paired with mothering is an even more poisonous concoction. We need to recognize that if the patriarchy can keep us fighting each other, we will never fight for change, and those who do will simply look crazy in their lone attempts. So in this, a society run solely by men will unfortunately never appraise the efforts of women because men do not see the bar being raised for themselves. Instead, without supporting female input, we will continue the endeavor to promote an unattainable myth of perfect motherhood that will push women further toward inevitable burnout and insanity.

Some of the invisible expectations placed on women include:

- that they possess a natural ability to be patient with children (Not *always* a female characteristic trait)
- that they are inherently able to expertly handle children
- that they are able to judge and direct age-appropriate activities for their children effortlessly without any requirement of learning.
- that they are able to maintain composure effortlessly, even during tantrums
- that they can cook and enjoy cooking for the family more than their partner
- that they are able to multitask and manage a successful career alongside parenting
- that they place a vested interest in the latest parenting strategies and their conformity to them
- that they are patient, empathetic, and hardly irritable
- that they should prioritize their partners and their children above themselves

The myth of motherhood is a tenet of our culture's most toxic ideologies. An ideal mother is rarely ever angry with her children. She is an archetype forged by sacrificial, relentless love. Our classics frame the perfect woman to be the kind that spends time at home—where she hones into a warm, homely haven that a man returns to after braving the dangerous world outside. Think of *The Odyssey* and the way that Odysseus was allowed to cheat on his wife and also explore the world for a period of 10 years, only to be welcomed home with open arms.

Penelope, in her love for her husband and her child, performs the duty that we all know too well. She is a dutiful wife, who fulfills herself in the significance she holds to the people around her. This symbol has not left us—even when we are considered to inhabit a time that exhibits the pinnacle of female freedom. How many women have you met who take pride in the way they prioritize their family over their own lives? It was not so long ago I raised my own hand. If my words seem a bit harsher than I intend them to be, know that you can love your husband and children with no diminishment when you choose to include yourself in the same level of care. I do not believe that my family embodies a single unit of life together— family is a layer. It took me a very long time to embrace this understanding that we are our own individuals, with rights to our own bodies, feelings, and interests. So as much as I love my family and the time that they occupy in my life, I cannot tell myself that I can use their lives as a buffer for my own sense of fulfillment. I need to have a purpose of my own, that doesn't relate to the ways in which I can provide for them— the words you read and the act of being able to write this book, are born from that.

A large portion of people reading this will disagree with me. You may find contention in the love that you hold for your family, and the many responsibilities that you carry in the name of that love you share. You may enjoy the routine that your family has given you, and the way that you have grown to become an irreplaceable part of their lives. You may find peace in the way in which the simplicity of caring for others contrasts with your professional life you may have not been originally called to; I did too in many ways. In these assumptions, I could still be on the wrong page—maybe not even coming close to the reasons behind your committed fulfillment. Each family is a universe of its own; and as an outsider, I can barely graze the surface of the depths to your icebergs.

However, even when you *do* fit the checklist of the ideal mom just as I did, the archetype is still damaging in the implications that it holds for your life. Despite how much you accomplish for your family, you will inevitably fall behind some other supermom in our world with unattainable expectations. You will still remain unthanked for your efforts, because you are simply expected to fulfill them. Even in the occasion of your exhaustion, you may find that you are not understood by those who look to you in search of perfection. The ideal does not exist. As mothers of the modern generation, we can reinvent the age-old tale and allow women to exist independent of these expectations. You have a right to conform or rebel knowing that all rules regarding womanhood and motherhood do not need to exist without change indefinitely. We are all grown adults, after all. The cultural ethics—which, in their bias and lack of logic outdate us and attempt to police our decisions—do not need a pillar. We are able to empower ourselves and the women around us in the domestic and professional life decisions that we all choose to make.

Sacrifices Made

Going back to my least favorite anecdote that I have with relation to my husband, part of the reason why him caring about the way he looks and matching his outfits to handsome perfection bothered me, is that it barely presents itself as anything out of the ordinary. Don't get me wrong! It's VERY nice to see him care about his appearance! But, he is not expected to —by societies standards— in the same way, and nobody gets offended if he doesn't. There is also something about a grubby man that can sometimes be adopted as attractive; queue five o'clock shadow. The privilege he and other men hold in being able to have the choice to leave the house in a peacoat and dress shoes, or crocs and a t shirt for the same activity astounds me. Women feel expected to dress up for any occasion more regularly. I have to at least fix my hair and put on makeup when I walk out the door and pretend like I 'Just woke up like this' even though I didn't. On the days when I *do* 'dress up', I have brought myself to a level of normal again. Often I get comments saying ' Wow, you look great! How do you manage it all?' And I wonder 'how should I respond to this question?'. Are women supposed to shrug and smile away our triumph at winning against the onslaught of a day that is crafted to defeat us? When someone asks me how I "manage," I am usually filled with confusion. First, I am not managing at all most of the time... just barely keeping my head above water. Secondly, am I not expected to manage? Do things really have to be at the extreme where it is an achievement for women to succeed in their mundane lives, and an embarrassment when they do not? Why is it only ever our stakes that are so dire? Why can I not be praised as successful in looking like I am working hard? It would be nice if the bigger the dark circles got under my eyes, the more recognition I got in public for my service as a mother. I will forever feel guilty for resenting the freedom that men are given as fathers, again taking on another weight that should not be mine. Mothers have to "manage," "make do," or magically "do it all." Fathers? They just exist. No one expects them to put in the same amount of effort that women are pushed into doing for their families today. Our society thinks fathers have enough on their plate unless it is a second helping of steak and potatoes while we keep being served more and more issues—as if we can never really be doing *enough*. In a viral Reddit community thread, mothers vented in anonymity about the unfair nature of parenting. Even when their partners attempt to give them "days off," they inevitably have to play the role of the mother to make up for their partner's inadequacies in parenting their child. On the days when women are allowed to sleep in, it is almost definite that she will have to face a mountain of chores that would make her regret her need for rest. Being a mother means constantly needing rest, and then hating yourself for having that ounce of human need. One mom complained about how her husband woke her up multiple times on her sleep-in days, to look for baby gear and ask her where the TV remote was. Her complaints were met with unanimous agreement. Another mom lamented how difficult it was to parent three children who were all under the age of three, considering it unreasonable to be expected to be pleasantly mannered with all the work that she constantly finds herself bombarded with. What these moms had in agreement was the fact that they were never expected to have actual *off* time. They were never given recreational time that they did not have to compensate for. They were never given any time with which they could enjoy detaching themselves from the identity of being a mother. As a mother myself, I find that I resonate with these women immensely, at my core.

Among the several sacrifices that we make in order to mother our children, we:

- experience the transformative effect that pregnancy has on our bodies
- hold the scars of childbirth, regardless of a C-section or vaginal birth—often, our hips and legs (and sometimes even the literal scars across our abdomens) carry the memories of our children's birthdays
- sacrifice our futures for the sake of our children's betterment
- have to make choices that remove, or detrimentally affect, our professional lives
- have to accept a novel part of ourselves that is more anxious, or prone to depressive episodes, than before
- begin to lose our energy to the infinite task of childcare
- make choices regarding our own meals in order to accommodate those of our children
- spend far more time tending to other people than we tend to ourselves

The list goes on, and yet—even in the peak of the sacrifices that we offer our families on a daily basis—these cries will still be the privileged complaints of women who can afford to live full lives after childbirth. In several parts of the world, people still lose their lives to giving birth.

One thousand women a day are caused to die because of pregnancy and childbirth. I use the term "caused to" because it is often the failure of their government and policy-makers that robs them of their lives. Eighty to ninety percent of these deaths are preventable (Turlington Burns, 2011). Isn't it a strange concept that the same birth that a woman does not think twice about in the Western world has to amount to a life or death situation elsewhere? Maternal safety and security, even in these extreme situations, still holds an unremarkably low spot in the list of priorities held by global health institutions. It is the failure of these institutions (and of us, as an ignorant public) that women have to suffer lifelong consequences for treatable issues that come with childbirth. *Obstetric fistula* is something you may not have heard of before. It is basically a life sentence to humiliation and isolation post-childbirth because of bladder (and sometimes renal) incontinence caused by long, obstructed labor experienced in the absence of professional medical care. The worst part about this condition is that it is entirely treatable. With enough awareness and funds directed their way, women would not have to fear for lives of shame and loneliness that are, unfortunately, out of their control in places this occurs such as sub-Saharan Africa, Asia, the Arab States region, Latin America and the Caribbean. After all, if they could help it, women would never have to live this way.

Is it not a shame that women still have to make these sacrifices in the modern age regardless of their countries? I do not include these figures as a means of diminishing the importance of your worries. The system has failed all of us. Many of us are unaware of the depth to which women have actually sacrificed themselves for a corrupt and uncaring society. Change needs to occur, urgently and insistently, to keep more of us from putting our lives on the line in order to have children. The births or pregnancies, no matter how early or oddly-timed they are, are not to blame; it is the system that fails to provide for these occasions.

It angers me, how much women are expected to sacrifice for a system that refuses to support us. Twenty-three percent of women consider the prospect of being a mother with a career to be an impossible task. No matter, a good percentage of us do not have the privilege of considering this an option—an impossible option, nonetheless. In addition, working mothers are also discriminated against in the workforce. We are seen as liabilities, who aren't ever as punctual or dedicated to our jobs as our childless counterparts. On average, it takes an appalling figure of four months of a working mother's wages to make up for that of a man's, and Fifty percent of our households today have working mothers as their breadwinners (Koziol, 2022). Our wage gap is so well defined that it subjugates us into different wealth classes. There is more to this number than simple male chauvinism. Women are often seen as somewhat of the leaky buckets of corporate industries. The knowledge that we sow is often reaped to a certain extent before we become mothers, who either quit the workforce altogether or start working part-time. In corporate terms, this translates to a wastage of resources—experience, skills, and labor squandered on people who don't hold onto full-time jobs. In strictly monetary terms, their logic makes sense. However, one of the many results of the transformative effects that the feminist revolution has had on our generation is that for the first time, working mothers make up the most educated demographic of the United States and Canada. This means that the workforce can't afford to lose us. We bring better skills and educational qualifications to the table than ever before—perhaps after finally being allowed to sit with the rest of the crowd.

The world has shifted beneath our feet—and while we lived our lives juggling between chores, telling ourselves that a task done half-ass'd was better than a task neglected, we were oblivious to our own value. As clichéd as this sounds, I find myself overwhelmed by this knowledge. For once, I do not belong to the lowest rung of the ladder that no one wants to be on. We have leverage. *Let that sink in.* You are an undeniable asset. They cannot afford to dismiss your applications anymore—not when you could offer so much to them. If you find yourself fuming at how everyone seems to be oblivious to this, as they still force you through the impossible cycle of tiring yourself to the bone before forcing yourself back onto your feet, you're not alone. If only the husbands, employers—or, even the babies—knew and vocalized how special you are, in the eyes of a capitalistic world, maybe you could you catch a break.

Here's the catch, dear Mama… they all do. It is why they hold you so tightly in the roles they demand from you. They do not want to compensate for what they can suck out of you—be it love, labor, or simply breastmilk. I will give the babies a break here. After all, they come from us! I will even give some husbands a break in the changing recognition as my husband has come to see. But, as the person in the middle of the tug-of-war, don't wait any longer to realize sometimes you need to call the shots. You do not have to be the one making all the sacrifices. You have done enough. From that first, frantic night, to when your toddler had goldfish crackers and tomato soup for lunch for the third time in a row, you have done enough. You have looked after others, in spite of how little you have looked after yourself. It's time that you start moving up the equality ladder without feeling guilty.

Not So Hypothetical: Questions to Ask Yourself

As you've reached the end of this chapter, think about the following questions:

- What are your thoughts on mommy influencing? Do you believe it adds to the pressure placed on the shoulders of mothers? Is it possible to share a social space where people can support all depictions of motherhood?
- Do mothers really have to "do it all?"
- What was the most difficult sacrifice that you have had to make regarding your motherhood?
- Where do you think change best starts for you?

CHAPTER 5

SHARING THE LOAD

"I am no longer accepting the things I cannot change.
I am changing the things I cannot accept."
—ANGELA DAVIS

In the times I found myself scrolling over other mom's posts in public groups online, I always found myself astonished at how frustratingly similar all of our problems seemed to be. I would see posts saying 'I wish my husband wanted to learn how to work the vacuum cleaner and actually empty it after' or questions like 'Does your husband know your babies formula ratio?'. More frequently, I would see a wishful statement such as 'I wish without having to tell him over and over, that he knew how important it was to apply the special cream I ordered after diaper changes to avoid serious rashes, because he knew that I had already spent too many hours and dollars testing out other creams that didn't work. Thanks for listening— just venting.' These mamas suffered similar ailments to mine, even if they were not exactly the same. They needed someone to take care of the grime on the bathroom tiles once in a while, or someone to wipe up the mac and cheese sauce quickly when it was painted on the highchair after lunch so it wouldn't stick and be impossible to scrub off before dinner. Maybe things wouldn't be as hard, and the workload would truly be fair if we could see ourselves as equals in certain aspects of parenting. And where areas of parenting fell to mothers needing to take on more—understanding and effort from her partner to uphold her seniority in those decisions could do wonders for their relationship. Our friends without kids reminded us that our problems were often trivial and fixable and to just relax and breathe and enjoy the moments. This is what we signed up for in having children after all… All we needed was a bit of communication improvement, or (if we could afford it) a housekeeper, and our problems would be miraculously solved. We could suddenly be like those influencer families that we stalked on social media. We would have our overnight oats and sip on our postpartum green smoothies and be done with this frantic phase of our lives. Of course, none of the childless friends talk about the repercussions and logistics of these instant solutions because they are not living in them, which makes it incredibly difficult to relate to.

It wasn't wrong in saying that we had problems with communication. Half of the domestic issues most of us moms had, were things that our husbands were blissfully unaware of. It did dawn on many of us I'm sure, from the very beginning, that we could tell our husbands. From the first day that my husband and I brought our son home, he carried our new baby boy up the stairs for me when I found myself too exhausted and sore from the c-section. I thought about telling him how difficult and overwhelming it all was, but he was awestruck by the moment, unaffected by the physicalities outside of a new human he could cradle in his arms. Back then, I couldn't imagine having any longevity to these new stresses. We are told how beautiful it all is, and not how to manage an equal load. I did everything naturally to nurture our child, and assumed he would too. I didn't realize that the struggles would always be changing and evolving. I didn't realize that I would end up juggling 2 kids with a 40-hour workweek with no support in the years to come, and I didn't realize that a pandemic was going to make life harder and more expensive to support a growing family. I didn't realize that most families would require a dual income just to get by. A day came, when I realized that I would have to be the one going to bed later, and getting up earlier than my husband—on a definitively daily basis— and my mind seemed to switch to defense mode. As someone who'd worked with time management professionally, I knew that the life we had planned for us as a family did not have real sustainability. My husband had the routine, and order that a male life had always possessed; get up, clock-in, clock-out, go home, relax. Our children had not transformed the way he lived his life in the same way that it had transformed mine. Our children were a part of his life; they were my entire life. If you have children yourself, I probably do not have to say more than that I was too busy—every day and for too much of my 24 hours—to be content with my lifestyle. However, I never said anything— at least in the beginning, I was too afraid to be the wife that let a baby come between us. Funnily enough, our baby did come between us. Visibly yet secretively (definitely yet not in verbal terms), the new addition to our lives appeared to add resentment to our relationship. Obviously though, our son was innocent of all of this. Nothing seemed to make sense.

We still:

- loved each other
- loved our baby boy
- were modern parents who did not think we believed in classic parenting roles for the most part

However, we also:

- conformed to the same classic parenting roles that applauded us
- didn't speak about everything that we considered taboo in a successful relationship

- aimed at being the perfect parent, knowing fully well that these were unattainable aspirations that often left us falling short of being the perfect partner.
- followed routines that ensured an unfair division of labor in the domestic front

Having a second child to re-spark *the wonderment* through the creation of life was blissful, but also short lived. The work that I would take up later on, did not ease any pressure. Even when I was in purely caveman terms, "earning my keep," I was doing too much for our family. It was not that my husband did not respect the work I did. He praised me for my commitment to my career when I wanted to return, and grew concerned about how my domestic life tended to stress and exhaust me. Still, when his concern translated to considering the ways in which he could help ease my workload, the efforts that he offered were not there for the long run you could say.

He would:

- make me morning tea one day for a gesture and not realize how continuing this would make such a huge difference to me if he kept it up!
- pick up the groceries, but need me to make the list, and go through the cupboards and the refrigerator. Sending him to the store more than once would be a no-go, so I would often find myself online ordering the things that I forgot to mention to him or just doing it myself to avoid the shame of forgetting.
- fold and put the laundry away all wrong
- wake me on the occasions that I could sleep in, as he didn't know where something was or how to do it

- inevitably leave me feeling like I was better off handling the housework, schedules, and mental and physical load all on my own.

What this eventually led to was my resentment at my workload, and angry mom rage at the way my world never seemed to support my lifestyle. As all problems have two sides though, I realize that I paved the way for some of the problems we faced by refusing to "say too much" because I feared that he would see me as a nag and we would fight. By facing each of my days like a battle I had to overcome on my own instead of simply setting up a proper system that he and I could both work around. By refusing to try some of the tips I studied and read because I was terrified of how failure would make me feel. And, by letting all the pressure build up on my shoulders, until I eventually cracked and blew up on him — and I mean BLEW UP!

It took getting to that point for me to invest in our future and our relationship and properly communicate and divide the unpaid domestic household labor within our home. I was stunned by the momentous nature of the change it brought about. It didn't happen overnight, but the peace it brought me was worth the long run that we took to save our sanities, and our love and respect for each-other. So, without further ado, let's delve into how you can approach managing your lifestyle—in terms of the physical and mental load that you take on—in a way that doesn't demand the full force of all your energy.

10 Tips on Sharing the Physical Load

I would like to take a moment to note that if you are in an unsafe relationship, these conversations may be much more difficult and perhaps dangerous. Please seek professional help before practising any suggestions if you feel you are, or could be in danger.

Discussing Why This Matters

Now that you've made the decision to implant change in your life, you need to bring the cards to the table. As familiar as listing your chores to your husband randomly on his off-hours may feel, you need to prioritize how sustainable your approach to your system is. Grab a piece of paper or a notebook, and write down that list of chores. Make it as organized as you want it to be. Remember, even chores that feel as minimal as loading the washer and dryer need to be accounted for. They take away your time and need to be made visible in order to count— so write down anything that takes up your time. Inform him of the ways you have too much to handle on your plate, and how you would appreciate it if he took some of the load off your shoulders. Tell your partner about how their help would benefit the both of you, and convey to them how much this would mean to you. Remember to be respectful of their time as much as you are of yours. If they work a full-time job, it may not be possible for you to get an equal split between the two of you if you are not working full time. Accept this and consider their input when you work out who does what. As old as the saying goes, communication *is* key. *Always* consider what your partner has to say about your needs with an open mind. *Always* be open to adjustments and remember to sustain dialogue about the things that matter to you. If you want to move forward, you will have to work through the nitty-gritty. Fear is an inch deep and a mile wide, so start the journey across it. You will get wet— but you are not going to drown. It's not going to stick on the first talk; it takes practise like anything.

Discuss Priorities With Your Partner

There may be days when your partner would want to hang out with his friends or family, and may not be as readily available to handle the kids. There may be days when you would rather go shopping with your crew or go to a yoga class than handle the dishes. Some of the commitments related to work, or maybe even those that involve self-interests, may not fit into the perfect schedule that you design for yourself and your family. Know that this is okay. You have a life outside of your family, just as your partner does. You do not need to avoid discussing the burden of handling a family just because it is commonly considered an unspoken part of raising children. It is only natural for the many needs, plans, and schedules that you plan for your family to coincide with other events that you find to be of significant importance in your life. Let yourself admit this and discuss priorities with your partner in a purely objective sense. Work out when someone would get their "me time" and set rules for how this time would be regulated. For instance, if your husband wakes you up on your quality Sunday sleep-in to ask you where the baby's shoes are, you can playfully punish this by removing 50 minutes from the hockey night that he shares with his friends at work. Similarly, if you keep calling during boys' night, or even texting about things he needs to take care of when he's home, you may have to face the consequence of losing a good chunk of your Thursday me time you chucked out for a much needed, completely uninterrupted bubble bath. These rules should be playful but taken seriously to meet both of your desired objectives. Think of how much of each activity you want in your life and discuss this with your partner. List down your needs, commitments, and other responsibilities. Now, let your household fill in the gaps seamlessly, as a responsibility that you will both respect and share equally. Your list can change and evolve over time and putting it together should be fun!

Lead With How You Feel

One of the most beneficial changes that I could bring into my relationship came with my decision to trust my feelings over what I thought I *should* be feeling. To clarify, much of the negativity about my marriage (which I often found myself dwelling on) was rooted in my habit of comparing my life to that of my friends' and the other people around me. There were certain unspoken no-gos that everybody seemed to be avoiding somehow, sometimes in the most forceful ways. For instance, none of my mom friends had their partners going out at night for drinks or hangouts on weekdays since becoming a parent. They had managed to reign their husbands in, *'surrendering'* you might say. Reflecting back, I desired control over my partner a little bit. I figured, if I was doing all the housework and the baby stuff, he should have the decency to let me boss him around just a little; this was subconscious. Things proved to be more complex than I had initially imagined them to be.

For starters, the times that my husband usually reserved for himself to relax or be social for after work were at home, gaming online with friends. He was physically there, but not in any other way. If the kids wanted something, it was still me to tend to them. This time was also the golden window that I often kept mentally reserved to handle the day's outstanding tasks for my work-from-home job that I always seemed to be stepping away from to do something for the kids. On the days I got the dishes done, the kids finally in bed, and the kitchen table clean, I would bring out all my devices for the next morning that I never brought out into the common space when my kids were awake. I found that there was little I wanted to do other than get some work done that I fell short on in the day. Having my husband at home, on these particular occasions when he was on day shift and not night shift, proved to be a bit of an inconvenience for me... and that hurts me to even say. Typing away while he played video games made me feel guilty because if I had denied him his leisure time only to ignore him for the rest of the night myself, it just didn't seem right. In my guilt, I would find myself trying to overcompensate for this denial by whipping him up some snacks and tea (while juggling work), Trying to sit down and talk about our days (pretending like this was quality time with each-other) with him still gaming and me answering work messages, and the whole circus was beginning to tire the both of us. So, we did what didn't initially feel intuitively better for the both of us. We did what was unconventional to do. Coming home from work, he would get his game time only after helping me with the remnants of the housework and kid duties, and I would get my peaceful work time in after the same. The kids would get to watch Scaredy Squirrel before bed in their room together, so that we could get 1 hour apart for our own stuff. Then we would both tackle bedtime and by the time we had them sleeping, we would both be somewhat recharged, and ready to actually spend time with each other a little before we had to sleep. Not every night worked out perfectly— as it rarely does with kids. Many nights we still lost, but the ones we gained made me feel human again, and I believe they helped him too!

Trust your feelings and speak from them. If you want your partner to make adjustments to their routine or lifestyle because of potential worries, anxieties, or fears, be honest with these feelings when you are trying to have meaningful conversations with them. Even if you feel silly about how trivial, pointless, or irrational your feelings may be, telling your partner about them will help you both arrive at the clarity you need in order to find a solution for your problem. If the sight of dirty laundry piling in your laundry bin makes you anxious, discuss this feeling with your partner. Even if you feel like you need to be able to work around feeling this way—or worse, toughen yourself up so that you don't worry about things like laundry—let your partner know about your anxiety. There may be times that your tight schedule may make loading and unloading the washing machine a bit of a hassle for you. Perhaps you have a tendency to forget about the clothes until it's the end of the day, when there's already so much more to do. Remember, while some tasks may seem unbearably heavy on you because you've already filled your plate, they might not actually be so for your partner, who may have a little space on theirs. The dirty laundry that triggers your feelings to spiral can be handled by a simple washing and unloading pattern followed before and after your husband's work hours. Instead of blaming him for not doing enough in the house, which will only be an indefinite accusation that they may find themselves helpless in solving, putting your feelings into words will allow you and your partner to delve into the intricacies of the issue you have found yourselves dealing with. Remember, you will never truly know until you try.

Anticipate Roadblocks

Having a plan, or a mental scheme, for how you want to go about your day can help you see the bigger picture that you want to focus on. Be conscious of reminding yourself that certain aspects of your life may be out of your immediate control. If you are tending to young, diarrhea-prone children under five, it is especially likely that you will hit a few (if not several) roadblocks along the way. Leave a little space in your work goals that you set for yourself, accommodating the attention that a child would potentially demand. With respect to your child's age and immunity, this period could range from twice a month to once a year. Give yourself enough time to breathe, so that sports practises, recitals, and competitions do not feel like burdens. Remember, even if you've got the entire school year jotted down to its last detail, there could always be cancellations and rescheduling. Do not let these obstacles get to you. Learn to take things in stride, even when they do not go the way that you planned them to. Your schedule and your partner's schedule, lifestyle, or work commitments may not always align with the mental script that you have set up for them. Learn to accept that this is okay. Anticipate the roadblocks. Doing so will help you better appreciate a clearer path and will also teach you the importance of backup plans, which cannot be exaggerated for their worth in the unadulterated world of young children. Note that backup plans should not be something only on your list. Create a backup plan together. Decide who becomes the default caregiver in which situation and why. Stick to it because if you both have deadlines to meet or meetings you cannot miss, these roadblocks will surely get between you two.

Agree on a Timetable

An early mistake that I experienced in sharing my physical load with the rest of the household had been underestimating the power of keeping records. I had read about how successful family timetables and chore lists became when they weren't simply things that were nagged at spouses and older children, but rather official duties that every member of the family was to be held accountable for. As much as I was all for establishing boundaries and finally getting rid of a bit of the load that had been weighing heavily on my shoulders, deep down I had not wanted to let go of my identity as the perfect mom figure. I feared that paperwork, even in the silly form of checklists and post-its, would simply be too much pressure for my family. I didn't want to be the helicopter mother who my kid would grow to complain about. I also didn't want to be the wife who packs a checklist of chores for her husband to do when he leaves for work in the morning. The myth of effortless, perfect mothering gets all of us, which is why it is considered to be one of the most negative falsities that we perpetuate as a society. After two weeks of secretly watching my husband forget his grocery lists, put the dishes away wrong, and suffer with the rather comically relatable belief that he was not cut out for this, I decided that I was going to have to brave the waters and help him feel welcome in the messy new roles he was taking on.

We scheduled a time, and I sat down with him for tea while Elsa sung in the background—courtesy of our daughter—and we had what I consider to be one of our most productive parenting discussions that afternoon.

While the specifics are bound to vary in accordance with the lifestyle led by your family, we found it helpful to:

- Categorize our time into fixed work hours, free time, and other commitments. Some of our friends found splitting the *other commitments* category into relevant subgroups helpful in giving them more clarity about their week, while others found this step a bit too time-consuming to be convenient in the long run. Always make a point of adjusting guidelines to fit your needs and preferences. What works for one family will be unlikely to work in the same way for another, so take care to work out the logistics with your loved ones.
- Make a point of working with our body clocks. I struggled in the morning, and my husband is always too exhausted from work to handle the kids at night. We found that we both don't enjoy being told what to do when we're on our "off hours" and we were more likely to get salty with each other. Hence, I take on half of the physical load at night: Making dinner, cleaning the toys up, giving the kids their nightly baths, and putting them to sleep. In return, my husband takes over mornings, always making sure to make the coffee, make breakfast for the kids, clean the kitchen, take care of the laundry, prepare a morning shower for our son if needed, and then drop him off at school when he can. The change was able to simplify the complex feelings of resentment that were left lingering in our relationship to a doable system that we both agreed on.

Avoid Gatekeeping

Your partner may have a different way of doing things than you do. They may follow a more carefree approach to parenting, or perhaps they may worry more about making the kids stick to a rigid schedule than you do. You may feel like you do the best job at certain aspects of their duties. Your pancakes may be fluffier than theirs, and you may make a point of never leaving the countertops dirty. I know you feel that you have different and legitimate reasons for interfering with their work. Your version of gatekeeping may vary from mine, which included criticizing how my husband considered it okay to once give our daughter gummy bears before dinner because she was being cute, and also interfering with mealtimes because I thought the kids were not really full from what he would prepare for them. This still does not negate the fact that gatekeeping, heedless of its form, is best avoided in family households. For one, it upends the purpose of splitting tasks. I wasn't really getting the peace of mind and quality sleep that I wanted when I was constantly busy nitpicking at how my husband worked around the house. Furthermore, gatekeeping may give your children a flawed impression of the nature of gendered parenting roles through the way you model household activities. I was a pro at gatekeeping to begin with. I have gotten much better at appreciating efforts made and realizing that rolling instead of folding t-shirts and putting them away is still getting them put into the drawers.

If you find it absolutely important to inform your partner about a change they need to include in their domestic chores, take measures to be respectful of them and their feelings in doing so. For instance, the gummy bear issue turned out to be pretty easy to solve. All it took was me admitting that I was anxious about introducing our daughter to too much sugar because our older child had developed a preference for sugar over his main meals when he had been younger and had dental issues. I had him put the kids to bed that night to see how it effected the routine and he got the point pretty quickly and is sure to keep an eye on the kids' sugar intake ever since. Now he's more particular with sugar than I am. I'm not saying that things will always work smoothly. Your partner may insist on the *wrong* brand of baby food, or always leave soapy splotches of water they forgot to wipe off after helping the kids wash their face. Trust your patience. Do not make the mistake of allowing them to use their supposed incompetence to get out of their chores. All forms of work account for someone's time and energy. Remember to respect this before you attempt to *correct* a task that your partner has already considered themselves to have fulfilled satisfactorily. It is okay to say something like "hey, my sleep shirt got all wet in the bathroom because of the water mess from the kids brushing their teeth. If they are super splashy, would you mind wiping it, or getting them to wipe it up to be courteous of others in the household? I will make sure to do the same on the days I'm helping them."

Touch Base Every Week

If your timetable is something that you plan on leaving alone, it may be likely that you will find it difficult to keep up with. The modern lives that we follow make it hard for our days, let alone months, to resemble each other exactly. You may take on projects that demand a different kind of work schedule than the one that you had been following when you originally made your schedule. Your partner may find it difficult to keep track of their new appointments along with their chore schedule. Expect this, and prepare for it. Whichever day of the week that both you and your partner agree on, go over your plans for the week ahead. Jot down any appointments, meetings, or commitments that either of you have scheduled for the week; we have a whiteboard on the fridge. Adjust your timetable accordingly, making arrangements for substitute childcare or household help for the days specified. If your partner's company or business requires them to frequently join unscheduled meetings, formulate a solid backup plan as we discussed earlier for such occasions. Take every roadblock that stands in your way as an opportunity for dialogue and productive communication. Before long, when your children no longer need such an intricate support system to help raise them, you will have successfully used the rough edges of the golden years to forge a timeless level of understanding with your partner.

Do Things Together

One of the land mines in our universe of parenting adventures had been our decision to often have one person run around doing chores while the other relaxed. In the beginning, I believed that the silly joy that I got from watching my husband mildly fail at elementary grade parenting would be enough to recharge my system. This was untrue. Things backfired when it turned out that all the childcare and housework would leave us with no time for each other. As clichéd as it sounds, the little competition that my husband and I had set up between us had become somewhat of a barrier between us. Within weeks of our tumultuous parenting war, both of us had become tired of how distant we were getting and we couldn't figure out how to bring ourselves closer without any resentment. As much as we loved our respective binge marathons on the rare occasions we could make them, we married each other for a reason outside of watching tv together, and the way we had decided to go about our household duties had burdened our relationship. One day I read something so incredibly obvious that gave me the hack that relieved us from our temporary separation.

This hack was a human tag team of sorts. Both of us doing our respective tasks together. By this principle, we adjusted our routines so that my moody morning self would have just a bit to do even in my drowsiness—as opposed to doing nothing, or doing it all. Similarly, my husband would no longer get to slack off entirely on his hours after work. He took over the lighter bits of my heavy night duties, just as I took to packing schoolbags. Essentially, we planned to lessen the load of the other person so we could cram in some time to chill together. It didn't match my read scenarios perfectly, but it didn't have to. What we agreed on fit perfectly (as close as you can get to perfection in the early child years) for the two of us, and we were satisfied with that. On another note, doing chores together will also help keep resident gatekeepers at bay, so that both of you are given an equal opportunity to tend to your household—and most importantly, connect with your children authentically. It became really fun to dance around each other on the loop of putting things away, both up on our feet, sometimes leaning in for a little kiss as we passed each other with full hands. We made jokes of the shared chivalry as we got to know each others preferences for order. We would congratulate each other for jobs well done! Complimenting each other for small tasks often helped light our spark. We were on the same team, winning or failing together. This alone improved our intimate desire for each other that was initially lost at the start of our parenting frustrations.

Flexibility

As pretty a picture it would be to pretend that the two-person village created by you and your partner will hold fort against every passing missile thrown your way, it is important to emphasize that success in interpersonal relationships is rooted in the participants' ability to compensate for each other. If your partner has a spontaneous meeting planned on your scheduled girls' night out for the week, you may have to consider sacrificing your recreational time for the sake of your partner because you would want them to do the same for you. Similarly, work and family commitments that you have on your plate may demand adjustments on your partner's side as well. Let these adjustments be the small acts of love that you owe each other. Do not make a big deal out of the actions you make for the sake of your partner. Even if your sacrifice amounts to a level of loss on your part, you need to let them know that you are willing to let things slide for their sake. Even within the frantic endeavor of counting your material tasks, obligations to your family, and responsibilities at your respective places of work, remember to hold tightly to the emotional bond that you have with your husband. Do not let your ego hinder your kindness. Your shared respect and kindness to each other will be the glue holding things together in the moments of panic. It may seem silly but for us, a simple 'I will make it up to you later' goes a long way!'

Keep Reevaluating

The world of parenting is an arena of change. What worked for you in the relative tranquility of the newborn days may not be the best solution for the comparative war zone of the "terrible two's" or in our case "treacherous three's". Your partner may have been your kids' favorite person to snuggle with when they were younger, confusing both of you when they suddenly decide to cling to you instead. When the occasion demands it, reevaluate your system and optimize it for better efficiency. Do not make the mistake of taking your reevaluations for failures. Raising children is a messy, often unpredictable challenge. Take the hits in stride. Go over the issues that come your way openly with your partner. If you find that both of you are out of options, you can always look for help from trusted friends. When our son started to feel left out when our daughter was born, I decided to let my husband handle her bath time routine so that I could give my son some quality *1-on-1* time that he needed. This meant that I could give him the cuddles that he craved for, and that our daughter—bundled warmly in her father's arms after wrapping up in a towel—would get some quality daddy time. The time our daughter spent with her dad in comparison to our son was much greater, and she has always sought his comfort and care more because of it. Remember, the recipe for a peaceful parenting journey lies in your ability to annotate between the guidelines set for you. So, be ready to experiment if you want to surprise yourself!

10 Tips on Sharing the Mental Load

I remember the last months of my first pregnancy as vividly as most mothers do. At the time, I had found myself consumed with nervous energy. I was anxious and uncomfortable and not getting a great nights sleep due to the size of my belly. I didn't know what motherhood felt like. My time had never been accounted for by anyone who needed to be fed directly from my breast, and the work that came with this and the task of transitioning to solid food. In contrast, my last days of childlessness feel strangely peaceful, if not empty. One of my vivid memories is researching what motherhood would feel like a few days before my due date. I had tracked my gestation periods every month following the growth cycle as it happened without mental efforts. I looked through Pinterest infographics on how to properly change a diaper, burp a newborn, and swaddle a receiving blanket. I stumbled across articles on how to treat mastitis, calm the scare of things constantly going wrong, and getting back to sleep when having to wake up six times each night. What my surface-level research made apparent to me was the concept of the "mom brain." At the time, I imagined it to be an overwhelming tide of hormones that would make me forget everything and possibly hate everyone. I wasn't too far off course. Motherhood *did* make me forgetful but I was lucky to not experience the anger and depression many mothers face postpartum. However, fluctuating hormones and the physical recovery that childbirth left for me, coupled with crushing anxiety had me falling behind from day one— or at least thinking I was.

    What Pinterest had left me unprepared for was a mental checklist that would grow to define the course of motherhood for me and I'm sure other moms as well. Suddenly, I was responsible for so much more than I had known, and the time these things took, didn't add up to leave me anytime in my day for the tasks that many Pinterest boards and mommy blogs painted as things that make you a good mother. My responsibilities overwhelmed my capacity to handle them on many days. This left me infinitely behind on all my *'plans'* for motherhood, which began to feel more like failure reminders than aspirations. I would be doomed to always be behind on the story books I wanted to read, the homemade baby food I was sure I would make, and the sensory learning crafts that looked fun online. I had no doubt that I would just slip these things into my everyday schedule and that moms who didn't do them were not *'trying hard enough'*. This phenomenon of overstocking myself left me forgetful and made my internal disappointment limitless. The mental load of motherhood is a term denoting the invisible mental tasks that a mother is expected to keep track of. Dividing your mental load is an important part of helping ease the overwhelming pressure that modern motherhood has amounted to.

Your mental load may look like this:

- keeping track of everyone's schedules— which includes knowing when and where every family member has to be at each time of the day
- remembering occasions of particular emotional value to your loved ones, so you can plan ahead for them (this may involve things such as highlighting dates like your mother-in-law's birthday, so you can make sure the kids send a hand made card; or planning a birthday party for each kid themed exactly how they wish for it to be—even tasks that carry joy have a mental weight of their own)
- deciding what to cook for the week and shopping to stock up on everything you need to bring your meal plans to existence (meal prep is my least favourite)
- deciding what to pack your children for school around allergies in the class even if they go against your kids dietary preferences.
- keeping track of medical appointments—depending on your child's age and your government's vaccination program, this may feature frequent visits to the doctor for things like immunity shots
- budgeting your needs according to your financial limitations—in some cases, many women have the added task of

- approximating the funds on the family's bank account when the couple fails to have transparent discussions about money
- scheduling shopping trips based on your children's growth spurts and replacing the clothes in their drawers.
- keeping a close eye on groceries and domestic supplies that need to be restocked, and replacing them when they do.

Discussing your mental load with your partner may be a significant way in which you can both make parenting work for your family. Remember, even if it feels like you have too much to negotiate with your partner about, the effort will go a long way in helping your family survive the rough tides of the early years.

Tip 1: Help Your Partner Understand Your Mental Load

Your partner needs to understand your mental load and how it makes you feel. They need to know this in precise terms, and in rational tones. The most frustrating thing about mental labor is that it is not as tangible as physical work. Back when we had still been navigating our second child's early days, nearly breaking under the tarmac of health anxieties post birth with our little girl and the onslaught of covid, I realized how vital it was for partners to resonate with our mental wavelength. I was constantly complaining to my husband about how I had too many loads of laundry to do that I barely had a way of keeping track of what needed to be done. As much as I wanted some help from him (and he had, apparently wanted to reach out to me), my frustrations had managed to distance me into a little bubble of my own. I kept panicking and spiraling, but I never told him what he actually needed to be doing.

What I mean by this is quite simple: Keep your partner attuned to the exact ways in which they may be able to help you. Give words to your gray blur of resentment. Route your frustration into its root causes and work your way out of it. Going through this process myself, I found catharsis in the way I was finally thinking of solutions to my problems instead of seeing them as hurdles that I had to tackle every day. It is so easy for women to get mad at men for not recognizing their privilege, when they don't even realize they did anything wrong. The work it takes to communicate will be worth it in the end.

Tip 2: Make a List of Your Mental Load

Even when your mental load may leave you more frazzled—maybe more irritable than you are used to—*try* not to take this out on your partner. I know this is asking a lot on some days. Yes, they *should* be doing more for you. Certain aspects of the excess you deal with on a daily basis may be a result of their failing to help you keep up with your work. Even so, accusation is a poor first step to take if you want to familiarize your partner with the world of chores that parenting demands. Speak to them when you both feel content. Make a point not to blame them, but to emphasize how much their help would mean to you. Write a list curtailing the variety of mental tasks that you often find yourself juggling. You could either present this to your husband or have a heart-to-heart with him, if your husband is more of an emotional thinker than an individual who works best with quantified work— mine works best with qualified work. You could even get creative with your work. A friend of mine discovered bullet journaling as a postpartum organizing hack. I love a good journal so I was all for hearing about it! What came as a way of keeping track of intervals between feeds, grew to be a hobby. Her mental load list is bulleted Instagram perfection; and she also enjoyed making it because it had an artistic element to it's creation. As a mother, I find myself craving the lost creativity in my life. If this is you, slip creativity into unsuspecting places… like listing your mental load. It can put the 'fun' in dysfunction. I also like mind maps, where I can tell what tasks go together and which ones lead to others. What translates well to a specific individual in labeled graphs, may be carried across to another in scheduled texts. Choose what works for you, and if one method doesn't work, don't give up! Try another.

As I always say, do what works for your family—just remember not to lose sight of your goal. Your bottom line should always be lessening your workload, so do not let your task scheduling become another job that you have to tick off on your checklist. Put your work on paper, but not so effortfully that your scheduling becomes a task of its own if you don't enjoy it. Begin as you mean to go on. Before you know it, you'll be a natural!

Tip. 3: Delegate Tasks

Just as you had done with your physical load, divide your mental load between yourself and your partner. If your children are old enough to do so, you can get them to pitch in as well, as a family activity. I really love incorporating a draw basket into our household. To do this, type out a list of chores on a piece of paper spaced apart about 1 square inch from each other. Print them and cut out the squares and laminate if you think they will get ruined. Throw them all in a basket and keep that basket at the front door. Each day your kids can pick a chore out of the basket that takes care of a physical load and it's paired mental load. For example, If your child is old enough to do so, make a card for the basket they can draw to pack their lunch box—you can set some ground rules to ensure they pack something nutritional along with their choice of snacks. Your kids can trade their cards in for something like screen time when they have completed the task. It's a win win! Depending on the age of your kids, you may have to take care of some of the mental load associated with the tasks, but it is a great start to learning. To level up with your partner, you can group your mental tasks according to the physical tasks. For instance, if your partner handles grocery shopping, let them be the one to keep track of your household's stock of groceries and toiletries. If they forget something, *do not* rush in to fix it— let them figure it out.

Tip 4: Play to Each Other's Strengths

Are you better at numbers than your more intuitive, emotionally-driven partner? Does your partner do an infinitely better job at coming up with nutritionally-balanced meal plans? Just as you split your physical tasks according to your preferences, you can delegate your mental load in accordance with your family dynamics. This removes the factor of having to drudge yourself through tasks you do not enjoy—a definite plus for your mental well-being! Talk to your partner about what you like and don't like doing and take the dreaded tasks off of each others hands if they don't bother you as much. These small gestures create more balance in your daily routines.

Tip 5: Take a Businesslike Approach

One of the most common complaints that women tended to bring up, was that gender roles and misogyny still made the division of labor in their households an endeavor that they had to push onto their uncooperative partners. Far from being a natural part of the work gone into maintaining a household, the splitting of tasks often fell on the shoulders of the woman, who was occasionally considered to be cumbersome in her insistence to be heard. In response to these complaints, women can disguise the chores into business tasks. After all, if men can be tricked by society into thinking that looking after their own family was submitting themselves to a subliminal feminine order of some kind, they can fall for a well-played game of pretend which gives them an opportunity to win which also boosts the ego, and helps you at the same time. Men are competitive creatures and are not hardwired for shame. Gamifying your tasks for a visual win or lose will light the fire in them to perform. Download a to-do list-themed app like Microsoft To-Do or Todoist - To-do list & Planner on both of your phones. Play swapsies and aptly fill in each other's schedules, taking care to set daily reminders that you can each compete at fulfilling. If your partner already uses a mode of their own to schedule their days, you could always incorporate their household checklist within this system. They may prefer to write down their tasks in their journal or prefer Google Calendars. Adjust accordingly. Our emphasis, at this point, has to be to present household duties as a nonnegotiable part of your partner's day.

Again, by redefining chores and being the core factor that drives your husband to the laundry room, you may still be filling the shoes of the hypothetical female figure who is always expected to be the manager of the household. However, there will be a friendly digital ping reminder on your side doing the nagging for you helping when we do not have the luxury of completely reinventing the culture that we are born into on a 360 degree turn. Even if your steps feel too effortful to be helpful, remember that you are only working through the essential systemization that will instill the habits that your household needs most direly. Once you've got your system in place and you no longer feel the need to double-check on your partner's grocery list, you may finally find that you can have the peace of mind that you truly deserve, and they will feel empowered with their new perfect score!

Tip 6: Be Flexible

Even when you've got your lives perfectly set on paper or in a scheduling app, there are several other factors that contribute to your mental load that you will have to accommodate. As a couple, time will show you that the mental pressure on each of you may not always be as equitable as your respective mental load lists. Certain things are out of our control, and—as frustrating as it is to anticipate the unpredictable—we need to be prepared. For instance, there may be more weighing on your mind than your child and your housework. If you live with an ailing parent (in contrast to your partner, whose own parents may be thankfully healthy for their age), it is likely that the care that you expend for them will take more of your mental load than you will care to write down on a piece of paper.

Similarly, if either of you are experiencing financial lows on the part of your business that require working overtime, you may need to consider this when you key in your plans for the day. Make a point of respecting the rights that you each owe to your friends, colleagues, and family—in their numerous birthdays, weddings, and other festivities that require their own levels of mental and physical planning. It is vital that you are both allowed room to breathe in the race that you maintain to keep up with for your children and your household. Remember to prioritize flexibility as a key concept for both of you. You have lives outside of parenting (or you should), and it is only fair that you allow yourself to make room for them. Stop and notice moments of stress for your partner and be compassionate. Tell them you notice there is something else on their mind and ask if there is anything you can do to help. Communicate to them if you need a grace day as well.

Tip 7: Set Up Your Home for Your Family, Not Your Guests

A few years ago I was looking through an past acquaintances insta feed she posted frequently on. I found myself shocked by how different her house looked from mine, but it wasn't because of the style or beautiful decor; she had two kids just like me now. What I was surprised by was that her home looked far more 'child-centric' than mine. Her kitchen had helper stepping stools and child accessible cupboards, I watched a video of her six-year-old retrieve his lunch box from his school bag and take out the Bentgo hard lunch box before pushing the soft bag into an open cupboard that had a space for it's storage. He opened his Bentgo and dumped the scraps into a small garbage in the kitchen instead of the big one under the sink that was harder to access. He then proceeded to carry the empty lunch box to the sink and dropped it in to be washed. Her son's school cupboard was carefully labeled, with writing marking exactly where the activity books went, reading books, and so on so that he could put his things away after school. To a kid, or conceivably a kindergarten classroom, their home probably looked awesome—being pretty easy to navigate. The caption read "he's such a good helper". My mind began to wander. Im sure there were toothbrushes hung from a little cup tacked to the wall in the bathroom and the ceiling shone with glow-in-the-dark dinosaurs in a playroom with a life size paper mâché tree in the corner stuffed with plush animals and a hundred age appropriate books. I took my eyes off my phone for a moment to look around at the overwhelming level of clutter my house seemed to be saturated in. I thought about how setting my house up in a more child centric way could save me a lot of stress —even without the imagined paper mâché tree. I wondered what it would be like to have my son dump his clothes in his own laundry basket. He preferred tossing it like a shot-put in no particular direction.

Depending on your level of comfort, attempt to make your home easier for your child to handle. Don't try and hide from the world that you live in a house with kids. Make them a part of it. It is 100% fine to incorporate the 'a child lives here' aesthetic to your perfect design. I really had to get over the fact that I didn't need the house that looked insta worthy #chrislovesjulia when I had two toddlers running around. Not that my house was that big or lavish, but I had been happy to accommodate a few kid-sized corners equipped with a timetable, and a designated space within my son's reach—that I could teach him to take care to unload his school books onto after school. There were several aspects of my preference that I didn't want to alter in order to ease my son into his domestic chores because design was so important to me. The little changes that *did* manifest in our home—from the effort to prioritize my son's needs over my father-in-laws assumed capacity to judge me, managed to ease my mental load significantly. I really struggled with having our fridge exploding with magnets and kids art, but they absolutely love making their creations and having a designated place to display them right away. It also saves me from cleaning papers off the table. As menial as some of these chores are for me, and some days I think it would be faster for me to just do it— it is one task off my own list and a fantastic learning moment for my kids who really love their new found independence. On some days, I still find that these little changes were all I needed to keep from feeling exhausted, and I can't help but smile with pride when I see my 3 year old daughter unloading the dishwasher to put her baby forks and spoons away in her own cutlery drawer.

Tip 8: Acknowledgment and Appreciation Are Important

The concept of praising men for their duties to their children and their households will earn me many eye-rolls from severely overworked mothers. They are *supposed* to be doing their duties, they would tell me. Do not place them on a pedestal, I would be warned. And I do agree. However, considering how worn out women feel by having to carry the invisible work that raising children demands, acknowledgment still appears to be an important element of how satisfied people feel by the work they put into certain aspects of their life. I am more of a traditional feminist and I don't agree with how modern feminism just expects change to suddenly appear out of no where because we deserve it. For example, I love making meals for people who praise how well I cooked, or simply acknowledge my efforts. I find it a chore to cook for anyone, who has a tendency to nitpick at the flavors I put in my meals in an un-constructive way. Similarly, my toddler took care to brush his teeth properly when we began to award his success with achievements from Sparkly (the Philips Sonicare for Kids app is amazing by the way). When by husband works out, I make a point of commenting on how fit all that working out makes him look. Reward systems, as pointless as they initially seem, have a tendency to work. Consider the most mundane parts of your chore list, such as taking out the trash or making sure that you fold the laundry neat enough so that your dresser doesn't look all that bad. These tasks often feel invisible in the light of the other tasks we do that overshadow them. Having someone take the time to appreciate the effort you've put into doing a satisfactory job would still feel good, even if you know that these tasks are unquestionably compulsory to you. There's something uniquely fulfilling about being seen. Even if it is just you catching your partner casually taking stock of your groceries—the effort that you put in to appreciate them will let them know that you are grateful for the care they have taken toward their duties. In the same way, making a habit of praising other members of the family will also help widen your perspective toward their contributions to the household. Make sure that the appreciation comes from a pure authentic place and is not pointing out that they have failed to do things in the past and that this is a nice change. You should see the look on my husbands face when I say "thank you for washing the dishes"—His posture changes, his chin goes up, and a small smile cracks on the left side of his face.

Tip 9: Decide What Your Glass Balls Are

In a speech delivered by Brian Dyson, the CEO of The Coca-Cola Company, priorities in life were compared to glass and rubber balls (Adib, 2021). According to Dyson, it was up to us to define what the hypothetical balls in our lives were made out of. Rubber balls could be juggled fearlessly. Even if we lost hold of our rubber balls, they would bounce back to us eventually. You could even put a pause on them. After all, rubber is strong. A few days on the back burner would do them no harm. However, glass balls are more fragile. Once dropped, you would be left with the excruciating task of picking up the shattered shards left behind. You can't juggle a glass ball. You need to hold tight to it.

Consider what the rubber balls are in your life. An analogy closer to our families understanding was my grandmother's china vs. the kids plates made of shatterproof plastic. I am very careful to keep our important dinnerware safe even when in use and I care for it when it's not on the table, not letting it collect dust. The toddler plates get thrown around. Rubber balls (or plastic plates) can be handled by your partner, or even by the kids—if they're old enough to do so. These could be the floors, the laundry, or the state of your living room. No one would truly mind living in a slightly messier home. Certain adults—and toddlers and pets—would hardly even notice. Yet, the absence of a glass ball is hard to go unnoticed. Your glass ball is comprised of you, your sanity, your well-being, Your family and friend relationships and the sense of content that you find in your life. Do not let yourself shatter under the weight of your mental load. Don't neglect your relationships, and your time that you appreciate with your loved ones because of the laundry. Pass on the rubber balls as much as you like, and don't forget to hold onto the things that really matter. When time has passed, the china becomes another family heirloom that you pass on… where as the plastic toddler plates? They almost always end up in getting thrown out or replaced.

Tip 10: Build a Support System Outside of Your Partner

One of the most important lessons that I learned when I moved homes to support my husband's job was that I had to avoid being dependent on him fully. By this, I do not mean that my husband is not a dependable person. On the contrary, he is definitely responsible, an extremely hard worker, and the perfect person to rely on. Before we met, I was completely independent though, and used to doing things on my own. Before moving back to Vancouver Island BC, I had a network of friends and family that wanted to be involved in our children's lives. I didn't want to completely fall into the position of making him feel the pressure of needing to take care of me when that was taken away by a new change of scenery. I learned that making a support system out of a single individual is beautiful in a marriage, but not so much in the world of parenting. It's too much pressure and expectation to balance on another individual, who is only as human as you are. Your partner is bound to run into spontaneous commitments, forgetfulness, or emergencies that will eventually leave you both without a backup plan. More importantly, your partner has their own mental and physical health to look after. These elements are too valuable for either of you to risk. This does not mean that you have to do everything by yourself. This book was born through my personal story of parenting almost completely alone— especially on the days where my husband was working 12 hour shifts 5 days a week. It is not sustainable or good for your mental health to do it all alone, and it is not worth trying to convince yourself that you are capable of raising children in isolation. Expand your support system, as much as you practically can. If the family isn't an option, think of friends, babysitters, day cares, or perhaps something like a cleaning service for your home if you can afford it. Hiring help may not be a reality for you, but welcome help where you can find it and do not suffer alone. The support system can quite literally be anything reliable that supports you. If you wish to find a community of other moms online, please join our 'Without a Village- Mothering Community' Facebook group. This group is a safe space to find your community online.

Sometimes the nudges we need are only little pushes in the right direction. Remember, making this work in a way that is achievable to both of you relies on your combined ability to put each other first and foremost. Keep sight of your goals together while also learning to let go. Just because you and your partner are *the parents* doesn't mean that you cannot get help. There is no competition. With time, we all do what we consider best for our families.

Case in point, I found one of the most achievable ways to split tasks with a loved one in Eve Rodsky's bestseller, *Fair Play* (Rodsky, 2019). Rodsky suggests to divvy up your domestic tasks in a card deck game that she designed. I am not affiliated with her product in any way, her book 'Fair Play' and associated game deck simply came out when I was in the editing phase of this book, and I wanted to add in how valuable it could be if you have the budget to support it. After all, there is no competition with helping mothers— we are all here to support each other. How it works is, when you decide to "play," you pick out the cards that will make up your deck for the day. So, the smaller the deck, the less you have to do. Part of the reason why fair play is so successful is that its method sets its limitations in a manageable manner. You do not have to chew more than you can swallow. Most importantly, you cannot decide to force food down your partner's throat either. As a couple, you decide which cards you have the energy to face and then split them between the two of you. As long as you've got a card in your hand, you are matched with a task that you have to fulfill. Rodsky stresses that your focus, in your game of fair play, does not have to be on getting the perfect 50:50. You could be satisfied with a 30:70, or a 60:40 between the two of you. What matters is that both you and your partner hold accountability for the tasks you take up. Whichever path you do decide to take to divide your domestic workload, remember that you need to focus on how achievable these tasks are to you. No schedule that manages to stress either of you deserves your time. Remember, all of this is for you to breathe a little easier so that both of you can have lives outside of your roles as parents.

10 Practical Tips for Single Moms

A disappointing finding for me had been how poorly our welfare system and society, in general, treat single mothers. Reports show that as of 2021, 80% of U.S. single-parent families were headed by single moms ("Single Mother Statistics," 2021). Unfortunately, even if this amounts to a significant minority at 23% single parent families across the U.S., this is still three times the share of children around the world at 7%

who are raised by single parents (United States Census Bureau, 2023). There needs to be systems made in place to provide single mothers what they truly deserve. Given how difficult enough it is to raise kids with a partner, being the sole caregiver for a growing child has to be a stressful endeavor. As per the experiences of friends and family, one of the greatest tasks that single mothers tend to struggle with is letting go of the need to compare their lives with other families. Things may be infinitely easier for you if there were another person in the picture to help with finances, or simply be with the kids—this is undeniable. Still, mulling a hypothetical *how*, or an unattainable *if*, will only hinder you in the path of enjoying the time you have with your children.

You may catch yourself stumbling under the overwhelming weight of the practicalities, the extracurriculars, the expenses, and the unending piles of laundry that need to be tended to. You may find yourself losing focus on those tender, irreplaceable moments of motherhood that our society fails you as it refuses to administer the support that it is necessitated to deliver. Wearing yourself thin to satisfy the role of being an extraordinary single mother to the children you love with all your heart doesn't compensate for the leeway that we all owe ourselves. As generic as it feels to write this, your children *will* grow up sooner than you will expect. There will be a day when you won't have to wash a poopy behind, or clean up the clutter that an afternoon play session warrants. Till then, do not lose sight of keeping your head above the water, and take these ten tips to help you even in the smallest of ways.

Tip 1: Order Groceries for Pickup

This sounds like an underwhelmingly simplistic tip, but ordering your groceries for pickup carries a few benefits unavailable to the more obvious delivery choices. For one, this forgoes an often hefty delivery fee. Ordering pickup also means that an employee hustling grocery bags into your trunk will assure that you do not have to unbuckle the sleeping toddler in your back seat in your attempts at actual grocery shopping. You could order your groceries online, and avoid the instance of tantrums for something off-budget or sugary they spotted in the checkout aisle (I say this wincing at the idea of my kids having a fit over Kinder Eggs strategically positioned on the lower shelf at the cash belt). Many of my friends swear by this tip, scheduling pickup times around the times that they already need to be out of the house to pick up a child from day care, or take them to karate. It is always easier to compare prices from the comfort of your home, where you would not have to worry about meal planning around sale items or doubling your work by flyer shopping at home and then going to the store to buy those items hoping they were all in stock.

Tip 2: Find a Playgroup

A playgroup can be a powerful way of teaching children how to make attachments to people that they do not meet on a day-to-day basis. Meaningful connections with chosen strangers can also assist with relieving you from issues with dependency that your child may have on you. On a lighter note, a playgroup will relieve both you and your child of the boredom that tends to frustrate us all. I myself met an amazing mom friend at the park down the road from my house in a fairly sleepy town and she is the thing that keeps me sane on the days the compile with difficult emotions. If you live in an area that supports it, there is a great app called *'Peanut'* that is like tinder for moms. You can create a profile and mutually agree to connect by both swiping on each other and opening up a conversation. Your profile can match you with mothers in your area and even those with children of the same age, and shared interests or hobbies.

Tip 3: Assign Chores

If they are old enough to, let your little one share a bit of your load. Maybe not your crippling anxiety or the unending list of bills that need to be paid on time, but you can involve them in the smaller things. You could start with tasks as obvious as stacking the toys back into their respective places or putting the shoes on the shelves. Let them be the ones to set the table, even if it means that you would have to head back to the kitchen to grab the spoon they forgot. Once they catch on and get into the rhythm, extend this to other chores, even creating exciting games out of them. *You* decide how to handle the load, so use every opportunity to lighten it. As the saying goes, 'work smart, not hard' and assigning chores is a smart move. With time, the tasks that they seem to be handling awkwardly will come naturally to them and they will develop important life skills that many teens today are quite honestly lacking and trying to make up for learning later in life.

Tip 4: Learn to Say No

Say no—this applies to both insistent children and pushy schoolteachers. You do not have to drain yourself of energy that you cannot afford to expend. Say no to extracurriculars that clash with your work schedule. Say no to toys that are out of the price range. Just—say—no. We want to do everything for our kids as mothers, but if you can pick a fair variety of yes's' that you know are your child's 'glass balls', don't stress to say no to the rest!

A single friend of mine admitted to experiencing an exclusive sense of guilt when things came down to disappointing her children. She wanted to compensate for the father that her children were missing by being both the "fun parent" and the "strict parent." She was well aware of how these roles contradicted each other. It was just that she didn't want her children to be affected by the cons of single-parenting, even when hiding said cons from her children would only amount to more work on her part. This feeling had extended itself to other aspects of her life too. She did not want to be defined by her role as her son's sole caretaker, so she burnt herself out trying to pretend that it didn't exhaust her to fulfill the duties expected of two people all on her own. With time, and many cathartic heartfelt self explorations, she realized that as satisfying it may be to beat the goals we set up for ourselves—it is vital that we learn to limit our aspirations in measure of their achievability. This meant giving leeway on some days where the kids refused to wear anything but pyjamas, and also holding the reigns on "no" firmly when the eldest found himself competing to be the friend who gave the best birthday gift at the party. It meant that my friend would have the opportunity to develop a healthier relationship with her journey in motherhood. The word "no" taught her children's teachers to be mindful of single mothers in planning events. "No" also taught her kids how not to expect the world to bend under their decisive commands.

While it would be nice to please all of those around you, the essential boundary that negation sets up will help you fortify the walls that you may require to protect your own sense of personal space, and also help the people around you to understand how essential it is to respect the boundaries of others.

If you are in a recently separated marriage, this may be more difficult because of expectations already paved from a two-parent household. If your child is old enough, have an honest conversation about what is important, and have your child list what is most important to them. Do your best to hold onto those things for them and you will learn without the need to discuss them over time as well. If you have managed to connect with a playgroup or other single moms, see if you can swap some of your loads to double the fun for your kids. Maybe you carpool host to baseball on Tuesday, and Friday your friend can be the host for swimming. Double pitching for birthday gifts or fundraiser bake sales can also lighten the financial and time commitment load. Give a gift from 2 best friends both signed on the card costing you each half. Double your cupcake load to cover another mum for the Christmas bake sale, and have them return the favour doubling their load for the spring fair.

Tip 5: Do Sleepover Exchanges

You deserve some nights for yourself, and so do the mom friends who you have around you. Once you deem your child to be old enough to do so, arrange for sleepover exchanges every now and then. Similar to what we discussed in the last tip with sharing your loads to give more breaks, pick a night when you feel like you can handle a few extra kids running around playing hide-and-seek in your household, and invite some of your kid's friends over. Remember not to go overboard with the whole event, there is no need to burden other parents with expectations for sleepover parties that go over their budgets if you cannot handle the cost of food and activities. The kids will love anything you throw at them. Their key interests will likely center on observing what kind of pyjamas their friends from school are wearing rather than picking through the assorted collection of fancy treats you picked up for them. Once you get the ball rolling, you will find other parents pitching in to host their own sleepovers. When they do, feel free to spend the night out with a friend of your own or even curl up in a sweater with the book you have been craving to delve into. You make the rules, so always remember to tweak them around to leave some space for yourself. You seriously deserve it and so do other single mums!

Tip 6: Create and Stick to a Routine

Moms thrive off routine. It's in our blood, right next to our ability to decipher what goes on in a TV show rendered mute by a screaming child. The act of creating routine is essentially creating order out of chaos. One could argue that the whole aspect of young life revolves around chaos— I know it does in my house most of the time. Even adults, with the self-regulatory skills that we learn to have perfected, are messy creatures. So, it is no surprise that our children don't come with all their needs sorted out. It takes time to learn. As a child-free friend once commented, 'kids are either dirty, hungry, need to sleep, or all three together', and from an outside perspective— it's fairly accurate. Routine, especially with regard to young children, provides the messiness with a semblance of order. My routine for much of my children's early years was completely chaotic. 4am wakeup for me while I helped my husband get ready for his 12 hour day-shift at the local paper mill, try to stay up and workout to stay healthy, but inevitably get called to action by a screaming toddler and I would end up tending to them and in their bed for the next 2 hours. Then second wake up. What time is it on my clock?—oh God! It's 8:30am… how is the kid still sleeping in now? Scramble for the rest of the day, rinse and repeat. A few years passed like that. Fast-forward to now— I do my best to label my routine as my blueprint, guiding me as I navigate my early mornings to hopeful early nights. I needed too when I started working from home with a 6am start time! I was already waking up at 4am, so I just needed to make those morning hours more predictable and take control of the messes a bit better. As Dr. Andrew Huberman states 'what we do habitually, makes up much of what we do entirely'. It can take as little as 18 days to adopt new habits. Imagine the positive benefits and time you will get back for forming good habits. Yes, sometimes my toddler will decide to sleep in a bit later than we are used to— she seems to take after her grandfather in that way, but our routine and the way our bodies are accustomed to it, will tell me what she will expect as she wakes up. Sticking to your routine, whatever it is lines up your dominoes for the rest of the day. Routine teaches my son that T.V. comes after the time that we all spend eating together at the table, doing crafts, or reading together. There are days when he insists on playing video games before reading, and I will cave if I have something important to do— but routines—even at their least productive moments, ensure that my children get their bare minimums done efficiently. A friend of mine says 'the drill sergeant comes out when the bed time routines start' and she corrals her boys as expected off to bed to sleep soundly like clockwork every night. I always admired how she said it like there was no other way. As a single or non-supported parent, you will live and breathe by your routine. To help me get started, I really liked using the *Habit* app and I still use it today.

Take this to be a special time in your life, where knowing the steps to the dance will still leave you oblivious to how things will eventually turn out. Know this and practice your routine anyway. Before long, you will be able to anticipate the sudden freestyle sequences that your kids tend to add to your choreography. Remember, it is better to know what you have to do for the day and manage to do it (albeit haphazardly), than spend all of your time wondering what you should do next and then wearing yourself out by anticipating the ways in which you will complete it. It adds a ton of extra mental work to not have a routine, so take a load off for yourself—The struggle in the beginning will pay off in the end, just as sleep training does.

Tip 7: Check for Local Mom Groups

No one will understand the experience of motherhood quite like a mother. I learned this the hard way like a right of passage as all mothers do. There's an acute legacy to womanhood, femininity, and the topsy-turvy experience of handling children while being the invisible pillars of society that men can never replicate. It is just the way things are. Similarly, your experience as a single mother may best be understood only by another single mother herself. In addition to the aid and conversation that may be of comfort to you, you may also find empowerment in how powerful a change you can enact in the lives of others. You see, what is difficult to establish on your own may be accomplished relatively easily by a group of strong-willed colleagues and friends. Check Facebook and take your chances, boldly and bravely. You never know which heights you will reach unless you care to try to manifest your desires. If you don't see a local mom group, consider creating one yourself! You've got nothing to loose and you and other mama's have so much to gain. You've got this, Mama. Go forth in full force!

Tip 8: Make Plans and Set Goals

Set aside time to sit down and plan your day. While you may feel like you have a world of chores to get done before you have time to sit down and organize your day, a large proportion of those chores are rooted in an unorganized schedule. These daily plans will intertwine with your habits we just discussed. At the beginning of your day, jot down what you need to plan to accomplish by the end of it. You don't need a Pinterest-worthy planner, or neat handwriting to do this but if you want to go that route, feel free! If you are more tech-savvy than you are comfortable with pen and paper, take your planning to a free mobile app. The key concept that we accomplish through these routines and schedules is thriving off limits. If you've got your work written down on paper and timed to your convenience, all you've got to do is *go with the flow*. What tends to hold most of us back is our fears of being wrong, of planning ideals that we will never truly live up to. Do not let these fears consume you. No one's watching, so you can test every trial and error that there is to this game until you get it right.

Start small and schedule the bare bones of your day. Write down the tasks that you've trained yourself to do quite naturally. Remember, even in their minute nature, they are also a part of the invisible load that mothers shoulder. Writing these down can help you build a sense of appreciation for yourself, as well as an awareness of your workload. Aim at making these effortless littles the thick of your to-do list. Achieve these tasks with pride, and then work on fleshing out your plans. With time, you can add in plans for self-care and both short-term and long-term goals. Motherhood doesn't always have to be about blindly making your way through the difficult years. You can have foresight, and you *can* hold onto your aspirations for the future. All you need is a little courage, and the willingness to try— trust me.

Tip 9: Plan Kid-Free Time

It's easy to become lost in the whirlwind of parenting. Suddenly you have got a whole other person to look after, and it seems like your own needs have become less important to you than they had before. Remember, you do not need me to tell you how valuable some time for yourself may be to you. I resonate deeply with the concept of craving for something—be it something as frivolous as ten minutes of an uninterrupted conversation with a friend on the phone or a subject deeply personal— like my need to find a greater connection to my long term life goals and inner self. Whichever your reasons and limitations are, you are not alone in this feminine struggle to move past the self-sacrificial version of motherhood that has been presented to us. You can and *will* have time for yourself. Close your eyes and say it like a mantra— *I have time for myself.* I know you are probably rolling your eyes right now thinking "easier said than done". I have been there going four years without more than two hours in a single day away from my son aside from the time that my daughter was born and I was in labour and delivery. That is 1458 days of constant care. It is what brought me to my breaking point. Schedule your kid-free time at regular intervals. These periods should not feel like vacations that you have to earn to deserve, but rather a routine part of your week that you frequent without associated feelings of guilt or liberation. Self-care should be a natural part of your week. Your body does not have to '*deserve*' random bouts of attention when you consider its suffering worth the additional excursion.

Make your kid-free time an affordable, perhaps occasionally luxurious, right that you owe yourself.

A few budget-friendly activities that you could do in your kid-free time include:

- reading for leisure
- soaking in a good bath, or simply standing in a hot shower with your eyes closed
- watching a rerun of your favorite television series
- enjoying a night out with friends
- Learning something new that you have always wanted to

You can utilize your kid-free time in whichever way suits you most appropriately. After all, it is time that you have entirely to yourself. Do not let the fear of judgment or the anxiety of trying new things get in your way! If you cannot make the time yourself and you can afford it, hire a sitter for your personal time. We fall accustom to saying yes to paid help only when it is on a work agenda. Learn to value that personal time to be more important (or at least as important) as the work meeting that could have been handled in an email.

Tip 10: Reach Out and Build a Support System

There goes a proverb that says it takes a village to raise a child. Unfortunately, our broken system leaves us stranded of our respective villages, forging a wave of overwhelmed mothers in its wake. Contrary to popular belief, the village does not only stand for a community of do-gooders who will happily watch over the kids for you while you kick in a good night's rest. While a community of this nature will surely be valuable, many of the villages we need, come from desires deeper than simple disconnection. You may need someone to listen to you vent about your child's picky eating habits. You may need someone to randomly pop over for tea and a quick chat on an odd afternoon when your children decided to leave you to your own devices. You may need company—people who celebrate with you, laugh with you, cry with you as you go through promotions, projectile vomits, or home videos that remind you of little moments that were magical or challenging. As an adult, you may have needs (both physical and emotional) that your baby's gummy smile cannot satisfy. You may crave adult conversation. You may yearn to be heard and responded to. It is perfectly normal to feel this way. Even when you are a mother, you cannot become an island.

Motherhood can become isolating, even all-consuming, in how it makes you the sole caretaker of another individual overnight. There is nothing quite like the responsibility that motherhood demands. This is why it is important that you build relationships with people outside of your household. In various cultures, it is quite normal for multiple families to live under one roof. What this achieves, quite efficiently, is the careful balance of caretaking and household duties. Perhaps you may not be able to summon your large and hypothetically supportive family to your household in a snap, but it is okay. Modern-day villages do not have to rely on blood. To the moms who have had to move away with their kids, as I have, and am on the brink of doing again, you can always find your village. My village came to me in the couple that frequented the same park that I did 3 days a week, my best friend that lives hundreds of miles away from me but still answers the phone on a whim to let me vent, or help me decide something new to make for dinner, and the mom communities that I found online. Of course there are always some bad apples in the groups. But, when I see negativity, instead of getting defensive, I really just want to ask 'Are you okay mama?'. My communities are not large, and I do not have the luxury of passing off my babies to any convenient substitutes whenever they are being fussy, or I have things that would be easier to accomplish without them—but my chosen village supports me when it counts in the ways that they can. I believe that is a considerable upgrade from my days in the darkest trench, pushing myself to burnout pretending like I could do it all on my own. You never know when you will need help. Having someone who you can rely on, undoubtedly, can come as a huge relief in those catastrophic emergency moments. Remember, you will not be the only person benefiting from these connections. Your children may also enjoy connecting with peers outside of a classroom context and close knit household. The people you will meet will likely treasure the change that you bring into their lives as well. It may be nerve-racking to stare in the face of all the possibilities where things could potentially go wrong, but tell yourself that you can't afford to think this way.

If you have the ability to travel with your kids, get out of your bubble and experience life with children outside of North America. America is an outlier from other developed countries when it comes to social support. You may be surprised to see your bills go down and your network grow if you have the flexibility to leave for a while. I am not suggesting fleeing your country, however consider how a change in perspective could influence your perception on what it means to be a mother in America.

You are brave. Summon the bravery of your motherhood as you feel your anxieties kick in. You and your family, may come to treasure the connections that you forge within your community. Most importantly, do not let your anxieties hold you back. Try your patience and reach out to those around you. With time—your village will come to you if your door is open and you are knocking on others.

Not So Hypothetical: Questions to Ask Yourself

- Why do you think modern-day parents still conform to the limitations of age-old gender roles?
- How do you think the concept of being an amicable partner affects how you parent and divide unpaid labor in a household with children?

- What do you believe are crucial points to having a successful dialogue with your partner?
- How have the stereotypical notions of femininity and speech affected the ways in which women appropriate their concerns to their partners? Do you consider saying 'too much' to be distasteful? If so, why do you think you feel this way?
- Do you think that a schedule or routine to organize your days would bring you some relief?
- What do you consider to be the glass balls or china plates in your life?

CHAPTER 6

BUILD YOUR CONFIDENCE

"Mother is a verb. It's something you do. Not just who you are."
—CHERYL LACEY DONOVAN

My first day of work stands as clear to me as my first day of school. I had dressed up for the occasion, but not to the extent that anyone would throw my efforts a second glance. To the outside world, I was simply a woman heading out to work; but on the inside, I was the woman who woke up early that morning to show up to work with perfectly styled hair that took me two hours to tame. I remember thinking I was going to take the professional world by storm. The feeling remains quite vivid, as it had soon been defeated by the reality of what the corporate world showed me in my first hour of official work.

Embarrassingly, humiliatingly (even when I believed that we had made a world of progress as women of the 21st century), I was still the one who was expected to run errands and *assist* other people in addition to my usual workload— But I volunteered as the eager new girl on the block. I wanted to show that I was dedicated and ready to take on anything. None of the men offered the same outreach of assistance outside of their hired job title. My meetings reminded me too much of my high school classroom, where the boys caused all the mischief and the girls sat back and did their work. Years later motherhood only added to this sense, with male gynaecologists, paediatricians, and partners holding the assumed privilege on far too many factors that left woman waiting on them. Even on the occasion that these men did have authority over me in their field of work, I found that my voice held a tendency to be overlooked because of its femininity. A man was always considered to be a better option: more trustworthy, less emotional, and—overall—a better choice to work with. Ironically enough, I found myself responding to this treatment without resentment. I always thought twice before I spoke at meetings. I missed work opportunities because I never believed I was good enough to apply for a raise until I met all conditions quite perfectly— that last one I still struggle with today.

Fast-forward 10 years and parenting was a whole other experience that I just couldn't teach myself to get the hang of before I was thrown into it. Either I was the authoritarian (who didn't let her kid have sweets) or I was the breezy parent who let her kid get away with anything. I have been told I'm being too hard and had eyes flared at me in the grocery store when I slapped my son's hand away from grabbing the straws hanging between the aisles for the sixteenth time after politely asking him not to— of course the other shoppers were blind to that part. I have been called a pussy, and been told I'm turning my son into a pussy for letting him lean into his emotions. As Ironically insulting that sounds— repeatedly and consequently, I felt like I didn't know what the 'right' thing to do was. A few hours of research, and years of watching other women sabotage themselves on both a professional and domestic basis, taught me that this strange lack of confidence is a phenomenon chronic to our sex and it lets people (and typically men) have the upper hand on us. Women are insecure about themselves—a weakness that both nature and nurture have instilled. Researchers have dubbed this effect to be called the "confidence gap," with findings showing that this perplexing sense of self-doubt holds damaging repercussions to our performance in day-to-day activities (Kay & Shipman, 2014). From lower pay grades to an inability to command respect from your own children, a lack of confidence may hold chilling consequences for you and your future. Turns out, it takes more than hard work and strong wills to compete with men on their own playing field— Women need to rewire their brain. On the brighter side of things, all is not lost. Even a subject as frustrating as a confidence gap can be closed with a changed perspective, and enough traditional feminist energy! Note that there are some major flaws in modern feminism. We are not overthrowing men in society like Xena warrior princess' swinging the pendulum too far in the other direction. We are building up equality and encouraging men to make room for our new found rights in a world built for them.

Join the Confidence Era

Of the many walls that keep women from thriving, the confidence gap is one of the least visible (yet more powerful) ones. Researchers found that if you are not confident about yourself, it takes very little to make you spiral into self-doubt, thereby leaving the task at hand in utter shambles. When I first read about this, I couldn't help but think of how unsurprising it was that an emotional issue was holding us back. Like most female leads in a badly written yet iconic 90's film— a majority of women are insecure. This wasn't really news, but it disappointed me to see reports confirm one of the attributes that women were often stereotyped for. It felt like being told that misogynistic men were right and that women *did* hold potential liabilities in the workplace. Thankfully, things proved to be more complex than my apparent dissatisfaction.

It's not that women are bad workers. From grade school to the corporate field, women are reported to be better workers than their more carefree male counterparts. Women are often more qualified than men, with more graduate degrees under their belts. In school-based research, girls were said to have better attention spans than boys, allowing them to concentrate on their work for longer periods of time. However, the reports also showed that the predispositions that gave women the upper hand in the classroom essentially pushed them back on the playing field. Women, apparently, considered preparation as a prerequisite for the tasks they attempted. Unless they felt absolutely qualified for every facet of a challenge, women were less likely to try at them. The logic works well on paper, but studies show that a level of risk-taking is necessitated in order for rapid-paced progress to actually take place. Men and boys were far more comfortable in their own skin than their female counterparts. They were more likely to overestimate themselves and take on challenges that were far above their pay grade. While this meant that they failed more frequently than women, it also meant that they allowed themselves to aspire for the occasional lucky draw. This intricate difference between the two sexes left women in positions that they were overqualified for, and men in higher positions that they, arguably, didn't deserve. Good job to the men, but what a difficult system for women to rise in.

Men and women are more similar than we are different, but research shows that we have varying dispositions toward affective skills. For instance, a woman is considered to be better at forging emotional connections and bonding with others than a man is. In contrast, a man may be a better risk-taker than a woman. While both defining aspects prove to be invaluable in the professional arena, risk-taking proves to be a crucial part of scaling the corporate ladder to success. To be fair, it's not only women who can be blamed for this phenomenon. Our gendered society reinforces female insecurity powerfully in the way that it condemns the notoriously career-driven woman for her "arrogance and selfishness," and the innocent yet self-assured classroom pet for being a "know-it-all." Our society taunts women by daring them to compete with men in their own playground, but holds the scales in a way that ensures their failure. Conditioned to hate herself, a woman doubts her capabilities and subjects herself to a lifetime of insecurities.

On a further note, it is not only the corporate scale that confidence plays a decisive role in. Self-doubt holds strong repercussions in both parenting and the maintenance of healthy relationships. It takes a solid self-image for an individual to be able to lead another person. This leaves little room for second-guessing.

Remember my struggle with choosing between authoritarian and more flexible parenting ideologies? My doubt in my capacity to make good parenting decisions translates to the self-image that I portray to my kids. Children are oddly perceptive, and the rule regarding no television before homework that I eventually gave into breaking every other night told them I was an inconsistent rule-maker. Tantrums that led to power struggles followed shortly, and I gave in to the belief that my kids were just too strong-willed for me to handle. Ironically enough, the truth was that I was being too weak-willed to carry out the goals that I'd set for myself.

Self-confidence can have a transformative effect on the way we love, parent, and carry on with our lives. Fortunately, the subject of confidence can be treated with a change in perspective and a few simple hacks— here are a few I have learned along the way.

Acknowledge Your Feelings

In listening to people talk about how women were always *too emotional* while we were growing up, many of us have grown to possess a tendency to bottle up our feelings. Even when postpartum made me feel like I was briefly bipolar but no where near what some women experience, I held onto the belief that I would not let myself crack under the weight of wildly fluctuating hormones mixed in with sleepless nights. While this ensured that I saved myself a few embarrassing tears in front of my husband (like when I chocked back crying because I just couldn't open the damn lid on the pasta jar), it also meant that he wouldn't know the level of hardship I found myself navigating. By suppressing my feelings, I spent far too long pretending things were okay and ignoring the root causes of my issues. My refusal to acknowledge my emotions meant that I would receive the help I needed far too late to be relieved about it, and that I had suffered for years on end to simply support the culture of shame that women continue to find themselves jostled by.

The version of motherhood that I had grown up watching on TV, and seeing at home, had been centered upon a skewed level of perfection. I would see my mother rushing to cook without even bothering to change her work clothes. It wasn't about the fact that she was tired, but that she wore her exhaustion and lack of time almost proudly. Mothers were supposed to be that way—selfless and angelic in how removed they were from mundane needs. Unfortunately, I internalized this worldview. I learned it from my mother. I will always cherish how hard she worked and how selfless she was and still is, but she deserved better. I told no one but my mother about how stressful it was to feed my son who does not like the taste of mixed textures and refused most foods. I forced myself to stay awake to cook and cover chores on the rare occasions that my son had a daytime nap, wanting nothing more but to lie down with him and put my tired body to rest because I knew I would pay for that nap when bedtime came. Motherhood, especially with my first, felt a lot like swallowing back my emotions because I felt as if I didn't have the time for them. It felt like stamping down emotional mayhem to make way for the sheer chaos that life had thrown at me. I lost myself in financial hardship, lack of support, and lack of security—I had lost myself to motherhood.

The prospect of letting my guard down, and allowing my husband and children to see my true self, terrified me. I didn't want to mix their more simplistic lives with the negativity that was consuming mine. In all of its self-sacrificial drama and heroic emotionlessness, reports now say that parents no longer need to limit their emotional selves for the audience of their children. Of course, this doesn't mean that it would be ideal for growing children to handle the extremes of the complexities that come with adult relationships. Researchers simply consider it more beneficial to foster authenticity in the relationships we create with our young. By their logic, letting your child see a pinch of the frustration that you may hold toward burning the grilled-cheese again may actually be beneficial to their social skills. Their exposure to your distress will teach them that accidents occur universally. Seeing you cry can teach your baby that other people cry too, and help them learn to shift perspectives between their own and those of yours, which acts as a powerful lesson in empathy. Again, it is important to stress how important it is to remove the stigma around letting your guard down in the vicinity of your kids, thereby relieving yourself of the stress of having to hold it together all the time. Lessons in empathy and self-expression do not, in any way, condone violent outbursts in their vicinity though.

The conversation about children and their emotional selves veers in between the lines of openness and sensibility. You can get angry at your kid for breaking your favorite mug. Emotionally blackmailing them and blaming them for other aspects of your life, though, is ill-advised behavior. The key point of this view is that emotions should not be off the table for family discussions. Instead, you could work on acknowledging and discussing them. Children mimic their parents and I have received comfort from my son and daughter after they hurt me with reckless unintentional childhood violence throwing a fist in a tantrum when they were mad. There was a time I burned my son's macaroni on the stove, and instead of being upset I ruined his lunch, he comforted me telling me it was okay, offering a loving hug because he saw how upset I was at myself.

Still, if you feel too disconnected from your own emotions and their respective sources, you may feel like you are ill-equipped to discuss feelings with your kids appropriately. In situations like this, try your best to give language and meaning to your emotions.

You may utilize the following exercise as an effective way to help acknowledge your emotions:

1. **Name your feelings:** Try your best to identify and label your emotions. For example, if you consider that the word "anger" best represents your emotions, write the word down on a piece of paper. It is important that you take care to be concise about the language that you use to represent your feelings. Hatred, for instance, can be argued to be distinctly different to anger. Reference a feelings wheel if you have a hard time identifying their names. My son brought one of these home from school and it is now up on our fridge.

2. **Put your emotions where they belong:** Part of learning to process emotions that overwhelm you is redefining the place that they hold in your life. Even when you feel like they have seized you at your worst, you have to be able to empower yourself to take control of them. As powerful as they may be, your whims are not infallible. Accept your feelings for what they are and position them to be removed from you. Imagine placing five feet between yourself and this feeling, which you consider to devastate you most intensely in your current state of mind. Detach yourself from this feeling, and let your heart observe it from an outsider's perspective.

3. **Articulate your emotions:** Allow yourself to give your emotions a structure appropriate to your liking. The key concept, in this context, is that you put yourself in charge of your emotions and the space you will allow them to occupy in your life. Think of the emotion that you have taken into consideration in definitive terms. Try specifying a color, size, and taste for this emotion.

4. **Reflect on your emotions:** Think about how you want yourself to be affected by this emotion. Consider the impact that the emotion has on your life, and how far you will allow it to influence the relationships you have with yourself and the people around you.

What observational exercises attempt to accomplish is re-centralizing the relationship between your emotions and yourself to a degree that you can perform mindful assessments of their impact in your life. Control will always be within your reach. Manifesting this control will involve empowering the relationship that you have with yourself. With time and practice, you will be able to exercise a degree of management and control over feelings—even in those moments where your emotions may threaten to devastate you. In order to feel confident in yourself and in the decisions that you make for both yourself and your family, you will need to be able to define those confusing feelings that overwhelm you. Redefine how you experience emotions. Sorting those abstract emotions into definitive terms will help you manage how far you will allow them to impact your life and your decisions. In turn, you will be able to direct this energy of being mindful and intentional about your feelings toward your children as well, allowing you to develop a more authentic emotional connection with them.

Have Realistic Expectations for Yourself

As most women eventually find out, the expectations that I had of motherhood before I had given birth varied greatly from those that I held onto postpartum. At first, I found myself ashamed by the sudden 360 of my life. Before Hudson, I had imagined myself replicating the lives of the women I had watched on TV shows and on social media. I had imagined myself cramming a side job of some sorts between a well-behaved and organically fed child, recreational interests, and an aesthetically pleasing mom life. I told myself that I would stick to my goals for myself. I told myself that I wouldn't be the mom panicking about childcare and an insatiable workload, only ending up eating my words when I made the decision to be a stay-at-home mother for the first five years of mom life. Looking back, it doesn't really seem like a big deal. I couldn't have foreseen how my husband would have to move for work, or the curveballs that would have completely thrown all of our plans off course. I couldn't have imagined how hard it was to be a mother mentally feeling like what we were providing was ever good enough. Still, things were never out of my hands. All it took was for me to establish what I expected from myself for me to be content with most aspects of my life again. Life does not have to be perfect for you to be happy even in the difficult times.

As individuals, it is important that we realize that there is only so much that we can do for ourselves. In writing this, I do not mean to convey any negative feelings. I'm sure that we *can* do it all, just like the women in the media who seem to be hustling with kids, ambitious professional aspirations, and the perfectly toned curves to go with them all. We *could* run the world in the best way— I truly believe it. Still, I stand firm in the belief that quality stands above the quantitative gains of hustling. Productivity can mean different things to different people. It is vital that we prioritize our mental health and our physical capacity to accomplish our goals when we create expectations for ourselves. At least in the frontiers of our personal lives, our expectations have to come from a place of self-awareness.

This does not necessarily mean that you have to be negative about your self-image, or that you should always underestimate yourself in order to protect your heart from the disappointment of failure. The mindset that you have for your own work, again, is entirely up to you. You choose how you want to feel about your workload. If the sense of fulfillment that you want to achieve on a day-to-day basis is better derived from a 70 to 30 percent split between your career and childcare duties, it is best that you implement this into your life, rather than fixating on the goals that other people appear to place for themselves. Similarly, if your best definition of a productive career comes from a level of commitment that can only be expected from a family with a child old enough to be dropped at kindergarten, your expectations for yourself can in turn be molded.

Identify your strengths and play to them. Set your expectations for your productivity with your priorities in check. In setting up realistic expectations for yourself, you will have to begin as you mean to go on.

Consider these following scenarios:

- If a day of work leaves you too physically exhausted for any form of recreational activities, your expectations for yourself may exceed your physical capacity to fulfill them.
- If tending to your infant's tantrums leaves you craving for rest, perhaps in the worrying form of numbness, you may need to talk to someone about a way of decreasing your mental load.

Remember to listen to your body, and work according to its comfort. Be gratuitous of your efforts and the achievements your body has granted you. A consciously appreciative quality toward yourself can help shape a healthy mentality toward productivity, which will henceforth have a transformative effect on the way that you view your workload.

The realistic quality of the expectations that you see for yourself must also extend to the other people in your life. Remember not to have any ideals about the state of your household or the "achievements" of those around you that strain your relationship with them. Discuss the expectations that you have with these people, and consider how these expectations will fit in with the expectations that they have for themselves. Keep in mind that in expecting things from your loved ones, you must be able to be respectful of their boundaries and also be conscious of the responsibilities that they hold toward their own lives. Be grateful for the favors they offer you, and be understanding of setbacks that come your way. Nothing, in parenting or in life in general, will come to you set in stone. You will have to make adjustments, bridging the gap between your internal aspirations toward your life to the tangible reality you find yourself dealing with.

Trust Your Mom-tuition

None of the blogs, parenting guides, or *mom-fluencers* I looked to before the birth of my first child proved to be helpful when I actually met him. Both the easiest (and most difficult) part of motherhood is the love. That first cry, that first touch of delicate skin on my fingertips—they were all that I needed to know that my love for him would take over me. To welcome a life you've birthed into the world is a strange feeling that engulfs you. I love him unconditionally. However, in those early days of sleepless nights and troubled insecurities, I found that I felt like I did not know *how* to love him. In hindsight, these words seem quite odd, in light of the wealth of material that proves a mother's love to be the most wholesome gift a child can receive. But, it is this same breed of branding that measures mothering by subjecting kids to inflexible standards.

When he loathed the sight of food outside of crackers and peaches (in spite of the pretty shapes I painstakingly cut into everything) I grew to hate the culture of shaming children on the highly subjective terms of "discipline" and "developmental milestones." The system gives no mercy to the mother who is unable to handle doing it all. Although this is less spoken about than the way mothers are dealt with, the cruelty that atypical children are shown resonates from the same roots of the illogical thinking that attempts to place all mothers in the same categories of prescriptive behavior.

My son experienced SPD and was struggling to process an overload of sensory input. He despised textured food, getting his hands dirty, or trying to feed himself. He was an unintentional night owl for months longer than other babies his age because we couldn't get him to eat dinner in less than 3 hours time. Under societal standards, he was labeled an undisciplined child from his earliest days. The system blanket blamed both me and his young self for the "failures" they assumed of him. The only way I could empower myself in the position I had been put in was to trust myself. To me, he was the most unique, talented, and extraordinary individual that I could have been blessed with raising. Only *I* knew the efforts that I exerted in mothering his struggles — which I didn't know were atypical at the time, until I had a daughter who was a normal eater that liked giving herself an avocado facial. I thought other parents were better at feeding than me, better at structure than I was, and overall something I was doing was 'wrong'. But, deep down I trusted I was doing everything right regardless of the output from him that I witnessed, and I put in more than double the efforts selflessly.

A friend once just *knew* her second pregnancy would be a baby boy. Another dreamt of her son a few months before his birth, sporting her late father's beautiful blonde curls and the baby blue T-shirt that she would gift him on his first birthday. You may have experienced similar occasions, where you and your children seemed to be inextricably bound by an invisible force—more supernatural than a cord of flesh. If it isn't the dreams and uncanny gender intuition, it is: the way you know what it was that caused your six-month-old's messy diarrhea episode, the way you know how to feed your daughter, the way you know when they are sleepy and not just mad, and the language of their love—which you navigate quite naturally in rhymes, giggles, and warm touches. Mom-tuition is the way a mother's instinct sometimes overrides the reasoning of other, equally qualified adults. It is the way in which your gut feeling proves to be more trustworthy than statistical proof and the conventions of parenting guides.

Upon discovering the name for it, I have been raving about *mom-ESP (extra-sensory perception)*. It is theorized that a mothers brain produces additional grey matter during pregnancy that could lead to this 'hyper-intuition'. The sheer amount of hours I spend with my child alone ranks me above all other competing adults in the field quite easily. No other person had been up past midnight with my children, so how could I possibly flatter myself about how powerful my intuition about their sleep schedule was? In logic, one would think if anyone else spent the same amount of time that I had tending to my kids, their intuition would surely overwhelm mine. To me, this thought only adds to the power of mom-tuition. No one said that mom-tuition is a mythical force owed to biological mothers, but it is fascinating and quite magical that we have the ability to connect to our children on a typically untapped frequency. Only a mother to my child could replicate the time, effort, and energy I poured into *knowing them* after the nine months of growing them.

Mom-tuition is a relationship that is honed by experience and curated by love. There have been countless times when I found my children's behavioral patterns to clash catastrophically with what was expected of them based on observations made of other children their age. Every time I found myself in such a situation, confused between my intuition and the parameters set for my children by experts, I found myself unable to pick a side. Like a classic first-timer, I pushed my gut to second place and went with what professionals seemed to think of the situation, warring against the voice of my body. What this often left behind was a panicked form of parenting, that resented the system for the way it treated my kids, and perpetuated self-directed hatred for the way it prevented me from being true to myself. We have gotten so far away from our natural parent instincts as spend countless hours pouring over monthly progression charts and 'what to expect' books.

One of the most empowering ways to regain control of the dynamic that you have with your children, regardless of how young they are, is to learn to trust yourself. Children are highly intuitive, especially on the emotional side of things. They will likely sense your uncertainty, just as you sense their first naughty streak. Be sure of yourself. If you feel like your child needs to tone down on their sweet intake, be firm on that rule about no sugar after dinner. Even when they begin to cry and war against the rules you set for them or give you puppy dog eyes, it is important that you practice consistency in their parenting. If you begin to doubt yourself and give in to their cries on day one, they will likely get even more difficult to handle on day two. Regardless of what other people say about you (and what your mind says about yourself in return), always look inward for guidance. Remember, *you* know your child the most. Turn to yourself, frequently and without fear, in order for your children to be able to trust your guidance. Even when it seems like no one seems to understand (or respect) your perspective toward parenting your kids, it is important that you stay true to your beliefs. Eventually, everything else will fall into place. It is important that you hold your ground on this until they do. A strong sense of self-trust will be something they learn from you.

Stop Worrying About the Opinions of Others

As a mother, I know how hard it is to navigate the realm of motherhood without the fear of being judged. My worrying comes naturally to me just like it did with my mum. My mother recently told me that only in her late adulthood, did she recognize that she struggled with high anxiety for so many years. My anxieties addressed all sorts of issues—from pressing deadlines, to issues as hypothetical as the potential flu. A bad mom habit that I had unconsciously reinforced over the years was a fear of falling short. I put so much effort into mothering and into making choices that ensured my children would have the most wholesome childhood possible, provided with the best food and the best upbringing, that I felt like I needed to foresee everything about it. When I felt that even in all my efforts, I was not living up to this expectation— I was a failure. Looking back, I can tell that I had skewed intentions about the whole ordeal. I was so focused on being the best at the superficial things, that I felt sure that any criticism or setback would break me and my children. I established backup plans for moments that didn't need them. My son's lunch box would even drain me of all my morning energy—it took so much effort to keep sending him food that would let his elementary school teacher know I was a mother who wanted her child to be well-fed while also catering to the class allergy restrictions, and an extremely picky eater. I aspired to be such a perfect mother that no one would dare bat an eyelash at how I raised my children. I would be miles ahead of everyone else. I would run so fast that no one would consider looking my way.

Eventually, as you would have already figured, my efforts got the best of me. I crashed and burned a little bit. My solution was to emulate the lives of other moms on my social feed. I would look at how they seemed to cook all three family's meals from scratch and drain myself in my attempts to bring this into practice without a single pizza night. I very easily ignored my ability to take into account that our lives were different. Maybe one mom did not have to balance her workload with the additional burden of a job. I would look at old friends with flat bellies and perky breasts, and struggle to incorporate an hour's workout into my already packed schedule, unconscious of how their unique lives and geographic locations provided them with more help, and their bottle fed children relieved them of the deflation of their bosom. By no means do I insinuate that these anecdotes are ways of proving how I was essentially tricked by my peers and my own mind. We only see what we want to see. From an outsider's perspective, I would probably look like the epitome of a composed mother as I dropped off my first child at school with a smile on my face and my daughter peacefully cradled in my right arm with her head on my shoulder. Our lives are all different, and what works for one of us will be an unlikely fit for another. We end up settling for the lives that we *can* keep up with, even if it means that our homes are messier and our meal plans less organic than we would prefer. An overt fixation with what other people might think leads to the eventual habit of living for other people. When I leave my priorities to my children, my health, and my relationship with my husband, I find my lifestyle a lot less cluttered than the one I used to lead worrying about what my kid's kindergarten teacher would potentially think. My habit of overthinking left me addicted to doing too much just for the sake of it, and giving into my anxiety when I wasn't contextually obligated to do so. If you've got a habit of worrying too much about what other people might think of you, it may be difficult to put it off on the first try. Mental habits are just like physical habits. Our bodies may be attuned to them, falling into their rhythm with effortless stride. In order to fight this, you need to redefine your body's mental habits.

You can attempt to redefine your body's mental habits by practicing the following:

- Make mental affirmations that appreciate the work you put into your day.
- Look to help those around you who seem to be struggling with their workload. This will help you appreciate how far you've come with your own workload, and also allow you to have a realistic perspective of how motherhood hits all of us differently—a need contrary to the perfectly glamorous lifestyles of the people you see on social media.
- Tell yourself that if anyone has something negative to say about your life, it is *their* attitude that needs to be fixed, not yours.
- Remind yourself that you cannot make your life fit another individual's perception of fulfillment. Work toward your own goals and find joy in completing them.
- If your lifestyle clashes with certain cultural values that burden you with more than you can handle on your plate, assess the practices against your priorities. Consider whether they benefit you physically or spiritually. Weigh in on factors like a possible fear of being judged for going against practices considered intrinsic to your community, and potential virtues on either side of the equation. Your actions do not always have to be emotionally charged. Be conscious of the emotional attachments that you make to your life choices. Stay objective, and focus on yourself. You do not have to prove anything to anyone.

- Even if the choices that you make for your family spark criticism or hard feelings from other people, always keep your priorities in check. You are only a peripheral part of the lives of the people around you. In spite of how guilty they may make you feel about your own decisions, it is likely that they will get over it soon enough. Still, if they don't, prepare yourself to accept this. All kinds of people may come up with negative things to say about you but, in the end, you will have to face the consequences of your life decisions on your own.
- Be selective of the advice that you decide to take from the people around you. Although we can all benefit from comparing notes with more experienced mothers, it is important to be cautious in using their practices in the context of our own lives. Think of it this way—while it may have suited your mother-in-law to make homemade, banana-flavored cereal for her baby in the early hours of the morning, the store-bought cereal would be a much better choice for you since you are too occupied with work to catch up on morning sleep. The differences in our lifestyles account for our varied approaches toward mothering—none of which makes either of us superior to the other. We are all different, and we must learn to appreciate the beauty in our diversities, rather than using them as a basis for our own sense of self-hatred.

Be Decisive

It is estimated that the average person makes about 35,000 decisions a day. Motherhood likely influences these decisions, possibly accounting for a good proportion that you have to make. From the birth of your child to the first time that you decide to step back into your office, motherhood is about the tough calls. Speaking from personal experience, decisiveness can definitely be a valuable game-changer. As a personality trait, it would mean that I would have spent far less time mulling over my actions and their consequences than I would have if I simply went ahead with what I'd planned to do. As a parenting skill, it would mean that my children would help me with the tough calls that parenting demands. It would mean that my children would know what poor decisions would mean for them, and the quick-fire quality of my decisiveness would put them off of anything too hair-raising. On a professional front, decisiveness it would mean that I would be candid about my compromises and firm about my refusals. It would mean that I dwindled less about the possibilities, and cut to the chase instead. Still, if it were so easy to be decisive, wouldn't we all be as sure-footed as we could possibly be?

If you catch yourself wondering how to be decisive, it is likely that you fall into the same category as I once had when my family grew. I was sporadic before kids, and I know that adding kids into the mix makes it hard, so if you have always had a hard time making decisions, here are a few tips. The best way to start becoming decisive is to simply *quit thinking about it!* Start implementing changes in your life that lean into a firm perspective. Begin with the little decisions. Make limiting the number of times you can rethink a decision relatively trivial to just two counts. The heavier life decisions that would require more cautiousness, you can grant yourself a greater number. Do not let yourself fall apart over decisions that would be of no immediate harm to your well-being. Wear whichever outfit you think is best for the day. Try out that new recipe, even if you are afraid your family won't like it. Strengthening your decision-making skills is all about teaching yourself to be confident, and not to worry about the consequences of your actions. Be brave in the face of change and be ready to start from the ground up again if you fail. As you train yourself to trust your instinct for the small fish, you will learn to keep your cool for the bigger ones. Familiarize yourself with the feeling of trusting your gut above all else. Before you know it, you will hold a strong command over your own decisions and also those of others, as they will turn to you as a trusted source of advice for the times when they feel like they need support in making their own choices. The key to learning a new skill is to believe in yourself. When it comes to decision-making, trust your ability to deal with any side of the coin. Once you've rationalized both sides of your argument, you will find that you have laid the groundwork for your quick thinking. Trust yourself and trust the process—with time, the rest will come naturally to you.

Find Your Tribe

Part of the powerful stride of a confident mom is her support system. For a long time, women like me (who traveled far from home due to responsibilities owed to their jobs or families) had little to no choice for a support system outside of their husbands. With immediate families out of the picture, and husbands occupied in the strenuous endeavor of their domestic jobs, homemaking was a load that women had to face on their own. As a partner to a husband who works 12-hour shifts, and a woman who lives several hundreds of miles away from her mother, I was left without many choices when it came to childcare. Before I had given birth to my son Hudson, I had not been acutely aware of how alone I would be in mothering my child. My husband's work, at the time was standard 9-5 but big life changes required us to move cities to small towns. This accounted for an often intolerable level of loneliness that I had not experienced before. A baby was a poor substitute for a conversational partner, regardless of how cute his gurgles could be. On the other hand, I couldn't really bother my husband all the time about how much I craved his company. The solution was depression, and the domestic duty of putting up with what I dubbed to be daily *pre-sleep-scream-fests*, or finding a mom tribe.

The modern age has proven to be quite abundant in providing the resources to connect with other people. As someone who has lived in both cities and also less populated townships, I consider myself quite well-versed in the basics of tribe-finding.

If you live in a city, consider these options:

- There might already be a ton of mom-centered niches for you to be a part of! You can look this up with your paediatrician if you want to find moms with kids your age, or do a Google search (be sure to specify your city in your search).
- You could join various activity groups targeted toward moms and young children. For instance, my mommy workout class gave me a great opportunity to connect with other moms with young children, and also strengthen my core after childbirth. I wouldn't have to worry about finding a babysitter to look after my little one. Plus, we were all too happy to cooperate with each other and take turns looking after each other's kids until our circuits were done.
- You could arrange playdates for your kids and connect with the moms along the way.
- You could schedule stroller walks with other mom friends, who have children young enough to fit into a kid stroller.
- You could schedule nights out with the moms you encounter—once you are comfortable with them.

Once I moved to small town Vancouver Island, I was pretty disappointed by how my tribe-hunting tactics seemed to fail me. There were barely any indoor activity clubs, let alone ones that accommodated mothers with children of the same age groups. My mom friends were out there, *somewhere*. I just needed to figure out a way to find them.

If you live in a sparsely populated area, consider these options:

- **Turn to church or other places of worship:** Most families tend to visit these places, and you would essentially have your routine meeting spot already scheduled for you. If you don't frequent your church often but are still part of the community, you could always meet your soon-to-be tribe members at church, and continue to schedule meetings with them elsewhere once you get the ball rolling.
- **Consider visiting parks to meet other moms:** Parks are an evidently good choice. Babies love nature, and playgrounds have a tendency to house many the panicked mom. I find good moms at parks!
- **Resort to online friendships:** Sure, you wouldn't be able to drop your kid off at a virtual friend's place, but the plethora of diverse mom groups online could provide you with the advice and emotional support that you need to shoulder your motherhood journey. My online mom's group provided me with quick medical advice when going to a doctor hadn't been an option for me, and uncountable parenting DIYs that helped keep my kids busy when I needed to get work done. With the onset of COVID-19, the few online friendships that I had with people proved to be extremely helpful in making me feel less lonely, and also letting me see how other people were tackling lockdown with kids in the equation. The 'Peanut' app introduced earlier in this book, has reportedly been considered useful in helping mothers find other parents to connect with.
- **Schools are a great resource:** Schools—yes, I know that this one will take a little more time than others (since you need to have a school-aged child to try this). However, school is arguably the

easiest space to hunt for parents with kids who are of the same age range as yours.

- **Look to niche-based groups:** You cannot expect these groups to house a uniform set of moms with one-year-olds as their primary membership, though. You might find a diverse range of individuals there instead, who have little to no interest in your children. Do not let this put you off. You might find them to be a refreshing source of change in your life. It may be rewarding to connect with people on subjects other than motherhood. Of course, this does not mean that you are ashamed of your kids either. Variety is important with mom connections. Go into the wild proudly, waving your mom card up in the air. If they are offended by this, you've likely dodged several bullets. If they look past this—as you will find several people who do—you stand a chance of gaining friendships that you may treasure in the future. Join the 'Without A Village Mothering Community' Facebook group before you put this book down— It's a great place to start!

On another note, it is important that you take care to nurture the friendships you stumble into. Trust me—your efforts will be worth it. Even if you aren't the most extroverted individual, you never know when you might need help. I met one of the few people I would come to refer to as a close friend on a casual day at the park. I asked her for her number because I had felt desperate for some form of connection at the time—and years later, we are still friends. The value of friendship doesn't always come in the help you can draw from them, but the company in friendship helps keep you off the edge of crazy when being a stay-at-home or working mom gets the best of you. I love my kids, but I would be lying if I said I didn't appreciate a conversation that didn't revolve around Gabby's Dollhouse, or most recently Bluey.

My best tips for nurturing your new friendships are:

- **Keep contact:** Make sure you have something beyond simple scheduling and meetups that keep you in contact. Send your friends memes, and check up on them occasionally.
- **Offer help:** Approach this pointer with caution and beware of sharks that will take advantage of you. If anyone is in need of help, you can reach out to them as a part of your annual 'Good Samaritan' checklist. Remember to always make sure to establish boundaries in a way that ensures you won't end up looking after your *friend's* kids every time they want to go grocery shopping or have a date night. This is not about expecting good in return from them, but simply laying the groundwork for relationships that are respectful of your personal boundaries.
- **Meet outside your obligations to your children:** A Mommy and Me class is a great way to ensure that you and your friends meet up every once in a while as your children learn how to keep their heads above the water; but once you lose the context to your meetups, you risk losing the connection that you worked so hard to maintain with them. The key to building friendships that go beyond the walls of the classroom is simply meeting outside of those walls. Whether it is the clichéd girl's night out or the more unconventional two-family game of monopoly, establish your friendships in a way that resonates with the essence of your personality, rather than simply limiting them to the company you seek in tending to childcare duties.

Friendships are never one-size-fits-all. You may have different, yet equally effective, ways of connecting with people. Whichever your approach is, it is important that you do not isolate yourself in looking after your children. You have a duty to yourself that you must tend to outside of your children. You need to look out for your own physical and mental health. You need to be able to find joy and fulfillment in your life. In order to do this, it is vital that you strengthen the sense of confidence you have in yourself. If a tribe of confident women and strong personal affirmations still leave you feeling vacant of the strength that you need to face the world, tell yourself that you will emanate confidence for the sake of your children. Kids learn from what they see around them. Exude confidence in the way you carry yourself, even if you don't necessarily feel this way most of the time. Treat yourself, your mind, body, and life the way you want your kids to as they grow up and have families of their own.

Not So Hypothetical: Questions to Ask Yourself

- How do you think the confidence gap has affected you and your life?
- What measures would you take, and consider beneficial to ensure that you gain more confidence in yourself?
- What would you consider a sustainable approach to setting goals?
- How does the concept of a feminine tribe fit into your life? How have you dealt with female friendships in the past, and how would you plan to approach them post-motherhood?

CHAPTER 7

TAKE CARE OF *YOU* FIRST

"Almost everything will work again if you unplug it for a few minutes, including you."

—ANNE LAMOTT

Why Self-Care Is Vital for Motherhood

Motherhood is joyful, just as it is tiresome. It's okay to say it. The words won't hurt you, or the kids. Parenting can be exhausting. It can become the most insidious drain of your time, and also your biggest trigger. As a mother of two, I am as much an expert on this subject as you are. My friend, a mother of 3, is sometimes similarly behind in the secret hacks of motherhood. Another friend tells me that it's not about quantity at all. By her logic, it doesn't matter how many kids you end up having if you are going to repeat the same parenting mistakes with each of them. The issue that has all three of us guiltily ashamed of ourselves is our evident lack of self-care. If we had more time for ourselves, we'd be much better at this than we are at present. With a bit of time to ourselves, we would do a much better job at mothering our kids. We would be kinder, more patient, and more capable of having more fun with our kids. And yet, none of us knew where we were expected to fit in self-care in our already cramped schedules. Can you relate to this?

The issue that most of us have with self-care, and how it is specifically marketed to moms, is how it is likened to luxury. While everyone has a little luxury every now and then, it isn't quite like a habit that you make a conscious attempt at following. How often have you been advised to have a night out with friends once a month, with the frequency of the event being a clear indicator of how it has to be *earned* to be a reality for you? In contrast, how often does someone tell you to let your partner look after the kids twice a week, till you finally went out and looked after yourself? People in our lives are not entirely to blame. There's a likely certainty that a concerned sibling or friend may have pointed out the importance of self-care to you on enough occasions, but you just hadn't wanted to really listen as you went over all the concerning *what ifs* as the primary mental and physical default member of the family.

Either way, I won't blame you here. Motherhood is a deeply subjective experience as I have said before. What comes to one person as second nature may be a lot harder for another, and there's nothing that can describe these beautiful idiosyncrasies in a way that is sincere enough to what they present to us in reality. Among all our differences, we mothers are bound by a curiously unadulterated love, which is an emotion so ruthless in its force that it leaves us expending ourselves in its name.

I will never forget the first days of my children's lives and how with tired eyes, I still scanned them for hours to know every inch of their bodies beautiful details. I will never forget the lightness of holding them, snuggled in the warmth of my arms. I can attest that the force of the love I have for my children does not come close to any of the emotions I have had for any other individuals in my life. I am sure you are the same. However, sometimes it is this very love that causes mothers to develop an unhealthy style of parenting. I was terrified of losing the unique beauty of the love that I had for my kids, so I was careful with the love I expended for myself. This comes to me as a *'classic-mom'* mistake. Self-sacrificial qualities look dazzling on paper, but what they inevitably lead to are crash-and-burn situations that leave us unable to care for our loved ones around us. Self-care should be a routine part of all our systems, irrespective of how cluttered they are. As natural as scrubbing your bathtub or picking up the needed cleaning supplies at the store, you should be invested in your bodies mental, physical, and socially motivated self-care. This stands impartial for the weeks when you are at your busiest, and also the days when you procrastinate on work and end up catching up on long-lost sleep.

Look after yourself consistently. Give your mind and body the kindness that it deserves. Even if doing so translates to taking a chore or two off your meticulous mom list, or earning a judgmental stare from members of the family, keep in mind that the peace you are fighting for will be worth your struggles. If you are looking for a way to raise your children without tuning into negative or resentful feelings, make self-care your key mantra. Remember, you *cannot* pour from an empty cup—and as a mother, you will definitely have your fair share of pouring to do. Always make sure that you've gotten your fill, and then tend to your little one. This may be a cliche saying, but it is repeated because it holds an incredible amount of truth for mothers. Your kids may be too young to understand the change in demeanor at the moment, but you will appreciate the sense of stability that it gives you and you can share with them how important it is to balance self care.

Physical Self-Care

Walking into the subject of physical self-care and motherhood is often like walking into a land mine— but it doesn't deserve to be that way. If you find yourself interested in the exaggerated amounts of mom-directed media elements like I do, you may have noticed how repeatedly bombarded we are by the image of a clammy woman in pyjamas with her hair in a messy bun. We are supposed to relate with that woman. That woman, in all her unkempt, exaggerated glory was supposed to represent the look of all moms. It wasn't that I was never a little clammy from one too many days not showered, or that I never got out of my night clothes first thing in the morning. Sometimes, I spent days in them. The fact that people were trying to normalize dishevelment as the symbol of motherhood put me off because I was tired of hearing people say 'I was beautiful before I had kids'— I myself said this. I was tired of people flaunting their lack of self-care as a symbol of the sacrifice they were making for their kids. Moms should look good *too*. We should take pride in our appearance—not because we are striving to compete with the megastar moms we may see on TV or social media, but because we need to be able to be confident in our own skin.

As easy as it would be to deny it, our appearance *does* affect how we see ourselves. After all, we are individuals of our own right before we are mothers—and our likelihood of appreciating aesthetic beauty in our surroundings means that we will find satisfaction in our beauty. I resorted to sweatpants and the mom bun on many occasions—this was a casual look that I resorted to quite frequently. However, making the image an emblem of motherhood feels undeniably harmful. One of the many things that I find problematic about the icon of the clammy, messy-bun woman is that in her popularity, it also seems like overloading women with work to the point where they are incapable of looking after themselves is becoming a casual reality.

Part of the reason why physical care has grown to become a taboo of sorts in our society is that it is often associated with frivolity. The mentality that places child-rearing above every other aspect of our lives, from our basic appearances to the food we decide to cook for dinner, often detriments our comfort for a hypothetical state of absolute adoration. Here's the catch: Even when women spend their days prioritizing their children's needs before their own needs, living on quick showers and the quickest hairdo, they may grow to foster resentment toward their kids for the facets of their lives they lose to child-rearing. The mentalities that *the kids always come first*, and *I barely have time for myself after giving birth*, often express the effects of overdue self-care sessions placed on the back burner. It's an elephant in the room to discuss, but it exist, and quite openly in Facebook groups dedicated to be a safe space for women who feel they regret having children because it took away their lives.

Mothers do not have to live this way. As much as you love your children, you need to love yourself. If this love is best conveyed in an intricate Dutch braid, so be it. If you consider yourself satisfied with a ponytail, then go for it. The focus of the physical care that you provide yourself does not have to mean looking like a supermodel on a daily basis. Rather, it is pushing a reality where you are allowed to present yourself in the way that you desire *even* when you are a mother. The roles you play firstly as an individual and then as a mother do not have to contradict each other. You are not doing your child any harm by taking the time to look after yourself. Wear the fun outfits with the wild patters if that is who you are! Even if you have the responsibility of raising your children, the bottom line is that your time is very much your own to decide how you want to be viewed by the world.

By looking to establish a routinely self-satisfying physical appearance, you will also be teaching your children the importance of looking after themselves. Children model the behavior that they see around them. You do not want them to be putting their own priorities—whether they revolve around children, assignments, or work—before the care that they owe their bodies. Making the upkeep of your physical appearance an element of your domestic routine that you take a pointed effort in maintaining will be a powerful way of reminding your children how important it is that they look out for themselves. The world is harsh in the expectations that it places on people in the name of productivity. The modern-day mom is simultaneously expected to be the best homemaker and the best career woman, when in reality these ideological terms prove to be poor tools for measuring our success. With time, these expectations will likely keep increasing in their weight. We do not have to accept either of these notions.

The physical self-care that you find appropriate for your lifestyle may be:

- taking the time to have a good shower *before* your partner heads to work
- incorporating hair and makeup rituals into your morning routine if you like that
- fitting in a workout session early in the morning—if you have early morning risers in your household you could always opt for physical activity like yoga or Zumba dancing, which you could do in the company of young children without risking any accidents, as you might do with a treadmill
- If you have a pet that needs walking, fit in a run or exercise routine with the task of getting the dog out. You will enjoy the shared exercise with your furry friend. But if this doesn't feel like self care to you—don't mix the two!

Among the physical self-care practices that I have managed to accumulate for myself over the years, if I could narrow down the habits (which I consider most essential for my mental well-being) they would be limited to drinking lemon water first thing in the morning, eating healthy, practicing a 5 minute meditation daily (usually in the a.m), Making my daily cup of matcha, and yoga or exercise rotations depending on how I feel. Focusing on your sleep as much as possible is also incredibly important. These habits make a sum of the struggles that I attempt at battling on a grassroots level, much more bearable. A poor diet, poor self-awareness, inflexibility, anxiety, and sleep deprivation will make just about every situation much worse. Food, water, a bit of self-conscious stretching, and sleeping may not be the most 'life-changing' solutions to the bigger elephants that tend to occupy our lives, but they can form important elements of our mental framework that will create big change over time. On a personal level, these habits were able to create enough change in my life that they triggered a chain reaction in my system that forced me out of my less-than-holistic lifestyle. They reminded me of how important it was for me to feel nourished by the life I was living, instead of simply moving forth with my responsibilities as if they were a part of my emotional baggage. While I did slip up with the occasional instant ramen (as most of us tend to do on our busy days), making a habit of consciously looking out for myself gave me a fresh perspective on the self-care that my body had been craving.

The following habits stood out to me as fundamental physical self-care hacks that made me fit in more comfortably with the nature of my life:

- **Drinking water first thing in the morning:** Research proves that dehydration often affects your mental performance detrimentally, causing a lack of focus which results in procrastination. Drinking water on an empty stomach may aid you in digesting your morning meal, and also help restrict your calories to healthy levels. Water is an essential nutrient. Our body cannot function without it. Having a decent amount of water in your system will help you stay alert throughout the day and apply enough attention to your priorities. On another note, this is also the easiest self-care habit that you can implement into your lifestyle. Even on the sick days when my youngest would keep me up at night, I mentally made a point of sitting down for a glass of water in the morning. Adding it to my habit tracker helped! On a physical level, it provided my body with the nutrients that it needed. In a more internal sense, it served to be a reminder of the space and care I needed to delegate to myself. If you are anything like I had been, and are anxious about how self-care may possibly grow to become another task to be checked off on your mental checklist, try making an early morning glass of lemon water the first physical self-care habit that you owe yourself. If adding lemon seems to tedious in the beginning, start with plain old natural H_2O. It takes no time and is the most cost-effective self-care habit that you could implement into your lifestyle.

- **Make a weekly menu:** If you're the person who cooks for your household, this may come to you as a lifesaver. If you are not, it could still account for a needed degree of positive change in your life. A weekly meal plan could help ensure that you—and the rest of your family—are getting a variety of nutritious food to fill your bellies. Running a consistent weekly menu aids us in reducing our food waste, saving our time, sustaining our healthy appetites, and also looking out for our bank accounts! What meal planning showed us was that a ton of money—and food—were wasted in the back-and-forths that we tended to make when it came to our meals. Now we were forced into meal planning the hard way moving from a city to a small town, but it was still a wake-up call. One of the best ways that I have seen people implement this physical self-care hack is by using a magnetic whiteboard on their refrigerator or a chalk board. The weekly menus would go up on the board every Sunday, and other family members were encouraged to utilize their erasable whiteboard markers or chalk to add their suggestions to it. What started off as an easy way to make sure that family dietary needs were being met turned into a collaborative family activity. This method—or your version of it—can also help you see the division of mental and physical labor when it comes to family meals. My neighbour shared with me that she would pull out the recipe books and each member of the family would pick one or two meals for the week. I love this approach also.

- **Practicing yoga:** As my go-to exercise in my kids' early years, yoga was one of the few physical excursions that I could take wherever I went. This factor proved to be quite essential to me, because my husband's job meant that we had moved multiple times before my son's first birthday. Simplistic in how it didn't require heavy machinery or force my postpartum body into anything that was beyond its capacity to handle, yoga helped me get back in shape without putting too much pressure on myself. The best thing about yoga was how inwardly oriented it was as an activity. It also allowed me to disconnect from the world around me and really focus on what my body was feeling. While my daughter uses the time to giggle at poses, upside down in her version of a downward dog, yoga gave me the lifelong skill of knowing how to relax when the tension of life got too tight. As a starter skill, I learned how to use my breathing as a form of meditation. I learned to focus on our breath, how cold or warm it felt, and envision its journey through my body, connecting this image with my consciousness and how I often take it for granted. In a world full of instant dopamine hits (owed to endless scrolls on social media), I believe that meditation stands to be a needed part of our lives. Our bodies, used to technology around all the time, makes us dependent on them. Don't let your phone be at odds with practicing mindfulness. The benefits that mindful activity holds for your physical and mental health outweigh the awkward frump that you will have to work past. Don't worry, patience and consistency will let your body do the work you need it to do.

- **Get more sleep:** This point will probably earn me some skepticism, but needs to be taken for its worth. You've been through it all. You have seen the appalling statistics. A month's less sleep than the rest of the world—truly the universe's unfair bargaining chip for our otherwise peaceful days with our impossibly tiny little ones. Moms average a poor five hours of sleep per night for the first year of their babies' lives (Kirkova, 2013). That's two to three hours less than the average sleeping hours expected of an adult. Your sleep needs to be a priority. While the average tot takes a little while to get used to sleeping through the night, they do hold a greater tendency to sneak in more naps than we do during the day. Take these opportunities to sleep off your exhaustion. While a regular nap may cost you more chores than you believe you can afford, you must attend to your sleep as a priority that you rank above your chores period. Adjustments to laundry days and a cyclical approach to domestic tasks may help you set a healthier perspective of your household labor, perhaps resulting in dramatic changes to the overall time that you spend on the upkeep of your household but it will not strip literal years off your lifespan like lack of sleep will. It is important to remember that your approach toward unpaid household labor is respective to your health and self-care needs. Although this does not bring you a "clean slate," on a daily basis you will likely feel rested enough to deal with your day with the sense of patience and kindness that it deserves much more frequently. So get on that couch and cat nap with the baby monitor next to you. I dare you!

I can't deny that some of these habits may seem off-putting or far fetched at first glance. Most of us are too worn out from our day-to-day workloads to even *think* of considering fitting in any more activities into our checklists. I get it. However, self-care—especially self-care that is physical in nature—is quick to show its results. These activities may fit a bit awkwardly into your otherwise family- and business-oriented lifestyle, but with time, they will come naturally to you. Part of the reason why most people feel self-care to be unnecessary is because it is considered to be a need that sits outside the familial spectrum. As moms, we tend to put our needs below those of the people we care for. We need to move past the cultural perspective that associates personal time with frivolity. Mental well-being won't stomp on your foot and demand cookies the way your three-year-old might decide to do, but it is not irrelevant to you in its silence. You need to sustain it in the same way that you tend to other aspects of your life, since a neglected mental landscape hardly amounts to good grounds which allow an attempt to sow the seeds of peace. Putting your mental health on the line means possibly placing the physical and mental health of your loved ones at risk due to your inevitable burnout.

The time that you spend on any of these activities is up to your preference, and the activities that you choose are up to your preference. If you find yourself satisfied with a daily five-minute session, stick to it. The key rule, in this context, is staying consistent.

Mental Self-Care

Moms are mentally overworked, Its practically an acronym— **M**entally **O**verworked **M**others. It is often a struggle to fully satisfy our individual needs on a day-to-day basis even though we seem to have the ability to cater to the needs of multiple people demands with an even greater level of mental commitment. As talented as mothers tend to be in fulfilling extraordinary mental tasks, we aren't superhuman. It's okay to admit it. We need to decompress, disconnect, and relax in the same way that our Netflix-binging counterparts do. Not throwing men under the bus here, but sit down with your partner and compare your T.V watch time. Most of you will see a trend. If not a resort to save our sanities, what mental self-care offers to mothers is an invaluable opportunity to be able to find relaxation in parenting. The mental self-care that you attribute to yourself should seek to satisfy your aspirations of creating a healthy connection with your most inward self, rejuvenating you in a way that cultivates your mental capacity to face the rest of the world. From simple 5-minute decompression exercises to 20 minutes of meditation, your definition of mental self-care will likely be honed with how far you've trained your mind and body to accommodate it in your life. For instance, 20 minutes of silence may seem like a waste of time to someone inexperienced with meditation, while a habitual meditator might find it difficult to move forward with their day in the absence of their usual 20 minutes or more. Regardless of the potential unfamiliarity that you may experience with mental self-care practices, mindful activities prove to be undeniably transformative in the beneficial change that they allow into the lives of their practitioners. From physical health benefits to a proven ability to make partners more understanding and cooperative with each other, several positive lifestyle changes await a changed mentality toward mental self-care.

In the most basic sense of the term, mental self-care activities are practices that attempt to accommodate our innermost selves. A buzzword that you might have seen being used with mindfulness is *intentionality*. Too much of our lives revolve around accidents. From the fickle moods of our fussy toddlers, to the random content that we decide to entertain ourselves with on social media, to the hour of day when we finally decide to crash on the couch—too many of our days are run by arbitrary aspects that are beyond our control.

What I appreciated most about incorporating mindful practices as a consistently recurrent part of my daily routine is how they taught me how to exercise more control over my lifestyle. In the past, I believed that I could only account for the most tangible aspects of my life—sad moods, anxiety, and frustration came to me like unexpected houseguests. I never knew what to do with myself when I was overwhelmed, always resorting to outbursts at my husband, or unhealthy coping mechanisms— Yes I'm talking about that glass of red wine I wish was never a part of the stereotypical motherhood club. Mindfulness taught me how to be aware of my psyche, and prepare myself for what was to come accordingly. It taught me how important it was to have control over my emotions, as it was often an inability to read myself that led to my worst spirals.

Top Mental Self-Care Habits

Decompress

Child-rearing is known to take more patience than a fair quantity of people deems manageable. Regardless, women often spend their days suppressing their surmounting emotions (the acute feelings of stress, rage, and helplessness that raising children often renders us with) to support the growth of their children. This is simply one of the many givens of parenting. As parents, we often have to push ourselves to be kinder and more understanding than we may otherwise have grown used to being. While this, in light of your child's mental welfare, is likely to be a worthwhile effort—in the long run, it is important that you treat yourself for your pains too. Most women find nighttime to be the best period to wind down and chill after a busy day of tending to their children. I make a point of finding the right balance, if possible, during the daytime as well. As I mentioned previously in this book, finding a routine was a must I came across too late. Don't suffer longer than you have to. even in the trying first month of feeding your little one, strive to implement routine in your life and your children's. Have a rough schedule for needs like food, wake times, and the potty after you have introduced these to your baby if you have a little one. Be more rigid about aspects like your child's morning and night routines, screen time, and the time they spend in the bathtub. Setting a schedule will help you make sense of your day and also help your child acclimate to a routine of their choice. Remember not to get too carried away with your schedule and to always make a point of splitting your parenting chores and responsibilities with your partner. Even if you can do everything on your own, you don't *have* to, and you shouldn't.

Think about your wind down time. As I mentioned, most people find it easiest to wind down after their kids are asleep or before they are to wake up. Pick one that suits you best and make sure not to waste your kid-free hours making up for chores that you couldn't get to while you were awake. In fact, ban them! Make yourself a self care jar (swear-jar style) and put five dollars in it every time you slip up. You deserve your rest and the muddy floor can wait until after you have prioritized yourself first. If you fill your jar, only spend it in treating yourself! If your floor is cleaner than your body, you need to change that. Establish the necessity of your rest time as a family ground rule and break into your free time without shame. A friend of mine loves to spend the hours after her son falls asleep watching reruns of The Office on her phone. Another spends her time on a rigorous night routine, filled with burning sage, jade rollers, and skincare essentials. There is never a set formula to your downtime except for your own preferences and the ways in which your body best feels rejuvenated. I like to remind myself that my downtime must include a compulsory aspect of guilt-free pleasure—and also nourishment. I get this from a rather ritualistic cup of matcha, and listening to an audiobook. Note, it is quite easy to slink back into toxic ideologies if you have a tendency toward them, aka comparing yourself to others as you toxically scroll instagram. I have watched countless women slip into "guilty pleasures," which inevitably leads to the loss of the whole concept of self-care itself. We are all human, and likely to be sucked into the harmful social narratives that take advantage of our insecurities. As a measure of self-awareness, I always re-assess my self-care habits against points I consider important to a successful self-care session.

As a self-care ethic, I often like to ask myself:

- Am I enjoying my self-care?
- Am I mimicking certain aesthetics or cultural practices at the expense of my comfort or convenience?
- Have I associated my free time with toxic guilt, that measures my leisure time under my assumptions of productivity?
- Are my self-care practices beneficial to me in the long run, or will they simply make me feel bad about myself?

Journal Your Gratitude

This one is fairly straightforward: practice thankfulness. Yes, the patriarchy is insufferable. We still suffer under the unfair division of wealth across communities. Racism is real, and mothers are almost universally taken for granted. Our world is short of several things in the realm of equality and progress. However, while the problematic policies of our universe are a very tangible reality that we must work toward undoing, it is important that we separate our feelings of disappointment for the system with a self-destructive quality of overgeneralizing negativity toward all aspects of life. We all have certain blessings in our lives that others do not. Making gratitude a conscious habit that you put effort into practicing daily will help you create a more optimistic perspective toward your life.

Why is this important? As a stark contrast to the edgier, yet undeniably more dangerous skepticism, optimism has been studied to have a more positive effect on people on a physical and psychological basis. Optimistic people are reported to lead longer lives, with less stress and stress-related health issues. Does this mean you have to be oblivious to the evident pain around you? Of course not. You can be self-aware in your gratitude. In being thankful for your blessings, you are not supposing that your world is perfect. What gratitude inspires, in its most specific and localized sense, is a conscious understanding of your privilege in relation to others—and also a rejuvenated need to lend aid to those who have less than you.

My pro-tip for practicing sincere gratitude on a daily basis relies on specifics and limitations. Firstly, write down five things about your life that you are grateful for on a daily basis. As a rule, you can set an upper and lower limit to your points if you feel too restricted by the number five (I keep my minimum to three points and my maximum to eight). Secondly, be as specific as you can in writing down these points. You don't want to slip into the habit of writing down a generically one-worded list on the daily. What I mean is, if you want to write about your gratitude for your health, try to be as specific as possible as to *why* you are thankful for it. Instead of simply writing down the word "health," you could practice specification by adding, "I am grateful for how my body is healthier than it had once been." Putting the words on paper instead of simply thinking about them inwardly will help them gain a level of tangibility. As a form of mini-journaling, a gratitude list will help you express yourself creatively without the pressure of having to write too much. Within days, you will be able to observe a range of different traits that you are grateful for and practice a deeper level of appreciation for the life that you lead. If you have a hard time putting this into play every day of the week, start with one and build up. My old office used to practise Grati-Tuesdays where we would share something we were grateful for when we came into work Tuesday mornings. Implement this into your weekly routine and build up from there.

Start Each Day on a Positive Note

Even if you are the world's worst morning person, make a point of starting your day in a way that fills you with joy. As a rule of thumb, I tend to end and begin my days with activities that I enjoy. As grateful as we are for our blessings and our children, our bodies also need some time to recharge and reset. Personally, cooking for my family and helping them with their needs is one of my most sincere love languages. However, remembering to direct some of this positive energy toward myself has had a transformative effect on how I began to see my days.

For instance, I switched from meandering toward the coffee machine and spending the first 15 minutes of my day judging people on social media, to beginning my mornings with a happy-lite habit. For the first few weeks, I couldn't do without my coffee—but I pushed it to at least 45 min after waking. I sit with my eyes closed in front of my happy light and feel the warmth and imagine being on a beach or somewhere that makes me happy. I am up before the sun rises, so this has become incredibly important to me. About a month in, I was successfully able to transform the habitual triple coffees that I had on my mornings into a sun-light and 1 savoured cup of coffee hobby that had a lesser degree of leaving me on edge for the rest of the day. It doesn't matter if you decide to wake up at 5 a.m. or get out of bed by 9 a.m. No one is pushing you to sacrifice any sleep or push yourself toward habits that come unnatural to you. Many people may not be comfortable about meditating first thing in the morning or trying out physical movement before their coffee. I have a tendency to fall asleep on my yoga mat when I try to do it laying down, so I sit up. A friend of mine found her early mornings to be the best hour for her to reconnect with God, and devote herself in prayer. This can be especially meaningful if you are dealing with grief. Whichever activity it is that you decide to dedicate your waking time to, keep your intentions toward fulfilling your interests. Everything else can wait for later.

Other ways that you can start your day positively include:

- **Stretching on your bed just after you wake up:** You can leave strenuous stretches and flexibility exercises for later—your focus, at this point, should be on starting your day in a way that pleases you. Reach up high and curl your toes, twist your ankles and wrists and arch your back.
- **Following a skincare or beauty routine first thing in the morning:** We all tend to feel better about ourselves when we look the part. Practicing five minutes of physical self-care may help you feel mentally prepared for the day ahead of you. I also started whitening my teeth with a gel pen, or white strips while I get ready.
- **Setting goals for the rest of your day or week:** Some of us like to exercise a bit of order in our chaotic lives before we delve into our days. If organizing your day helps you mentally prepare for it, you can always start your day with your planner, planner app or method of choice.
- **Spreading joy, in any way possible:** Your first act of peace in the morning may be as simple as fishing for a funny meme to send your group chat—or even a more serious action, like sincerely telling a loved one how much you appreciate their presence in your life. The key notion of this tip is finding a sense of satisfaction in your ability to spread joy to the people around you. You may have experienced this before. If you meet someone who is a natural 'joy spreader' you will find them to be infectious.
- **Planning an entertaining activity for the end of the day:** A fun way of positively motivating yourself for the day ahead of you is incorporating something to look forward to at the end of your domestic schedule. You can pick from a range of activities such as family quiz nights, movie nights, or girls' nights. Be

ambitious with your choices. Your happiness is the most important thing here.

Practice Meditation

In spite of how busy you may be, developing a deeper connection with your mind and body is vital in helping you overcome stress and the fatigue it is capable of inducing. Anyone who has experienced bodily aches or anxiety knows how easy it is to feel burdened by issues that are beyond our control. With the element of motherhood added into the equation, it is easy to feel weighed down by yourself and to fall into a line of thinking that questions your worth with regard to your capability to manage your domestic responsibilities.

During the early days of my son's life, when I had been overwhelmed by the sudden onset of maternal duties, I remember feeling like my anxiety had a presence that I would always have to push myself to ignore if I planned on focusing. Our minds have a quality of wearing us down when we do push ourselves past our mental limits, and especially when a little humans life is the centre of that anxiety. Just as our muscles tire with strain and overwork, our minds have certain limitations that we may find difficult to transgress beyond. Part of the reason that we struggle so much with our responsibilities is because the connectivity and presence demanded by the modern world can overwhelm our capacity to manage stress. The fact that you may be prone to stress doesn't mean that you have to deny yourself productivity or work that you feel entitled to provide yourself with—it just means that you have to develop a better relationship with your mind and your inner thoughts. Meditation can be effective in achieving this, as it teaches you to look past distractions and work on bettering the relationship that you have with your mind and body.

Your first attempts at meditation don't have to require much of you, with the exception of your sincerity and consistency in practice. To incorporate productive meditation sessions into your daily routine, you should:

- **Pick a location that you consider to be free of distractions:** If you find this difficult to manage with children, try your best to minimize sonorous distractions around you. Turn off loud toys, lower the volume of the television or turn it off, and switch your phone's ringer to silent mode. White noise can also be used to drown out auditory distractions. Because mothers live in chaotically overstimulated environments, I find early morning or late evening the best time to meditate regardless of your location, these hours tend to be less distracting.

- **Aim for achievable goals:** Do not start your first meditation session with a whopping 20 minutes of silence! Even 5 minutes of meditation can do wonders for your sense of spiritual well-being. Don't put too much pressure on yourself to meet unreasonable goals.

- **Stretch:** Work out those kinks and knots in your arms and legs before you sit still on your yoga mat or cushion. Your first time will always be harder than you think, so prepare for it! Wiggle your toes, become aware of the tightness and tensions you may hold on one side of your body. Take a deep breath and try and relax those tensions before you begin.

- **Dress comfortably and let go of expectation:** You do not need expensive stretch pants or even a thick yoga mat to build a successful meditation habit. Wear comfortable clothing of your preference —even pyjamas work! I like loose linen. Whichever you choose, remember to be comfortable with your choices and to refine your habit as you go. Practise in a way that is directed toward your own self-satisfaction.

- **Lean in, clear your mind, and focus on your breathing:** The goal of meditation is actually quite simple: blocking off the rest of the world and letting your mind be blank for an extended period of time. It is okay if your mind wanders. Try to be aware of your reckless thoughts running away from you and pull them back in, telling your mind to recenter much like you would re-centre a GPS system back to 'you are here'. Use your breath to help you stay consistent, being conscious of the air flowing in and out of your body as you inhale and exhale.
- **Practice consistency:** Once you've made it through a single session, make meditation a habit that you stick to consistently. Some days will be shorter and some longer, but the importance is in showing up. Consider a guided meditation on an app like 'Calm' to keep you on track and excited about building your consistency.

Disconnect!

Addiction to screen time is real, and not only a problem exclusive to your toddler. Digital detox is a powerful way of regaining control of your mental habits. Even if you feel like a tendency to scroll through your timeline is a habit that you can cut yourself some slack with, studies have shown digital detoxes to have a restorative effect on the minds and bodies of tech addicts. Whether you are aware of it or have not given it much thought, our screens tend to suck away our time. Based on statistics made in 2022, the time that we spend on our screens roughly averages 3 hours and 15 minutes a day (Howarth, 2023). With technology growing more interactive and integrated with modern-day lifestyles, time is likely to only fast-track our descent into addiction. After all, if we are going to expect our children to practice restraint with their screen time, we need to show them a good example. Your screen (and the blue light it radiates) causes an addiction to overloading your system with the information it feeds you, but it also acts as a driving cause for sleep deprivation. The wavelength of blue light has been observed to have a quality of interfering with our body's circadian cycle—the natural bodily clock that has most of us sleeping at night, and awake during the day. This results in sleep issues that account for more fatigue and weariness in our waking hours. Sleep aside, the most popular applications that people tend to use on their phones have a quality of promoting mindlessness through the way in which its algorithms present us with content that is motivated to spark a dopamine thrill. While dopamine hits feel nice, repeated exposure reinforces a mentality that seeks pleasure that is instantaneous in nature, possibly affecting our ability to enjoy and focus on other elements of our lives.

To put the research into more relatable terms—a few hours without your cell phone might assure you of a sense of tranquility, but adding in several more may heighten the sense that you are "missing out" on certain things that you need to catch up on. The urge to check your emails, or refresh your timeline, may also translate to a similar degree of addiction as that subtle FOMO syndrome that lives integrated with technology tends to induce us with. So can we undo all of this? We need our phones, as a means of conveniently connecting with our loved ones and staying up-to-date on our social and professional calendars and investments, but practicing awareness and conscious limitations can help with managing our screen time to an achievable level. It can help us focus on self-growth and connecting with our loved ones in place of mindlessly spending time on our devices.

My tips for a manageable level of unplugging in a family context are:

- **Delegate screen-free places in your home:** Bedrooms, bathrooms, and dining areas may be considered strictly off-limits. A designated screen time room can also help with this, as long as you place restrictions on how long family members are allowed to spend their time there. Make a point of adhering to the rules that you set for your family, to help inspire them to follow. If you want to bump up the challenge, you can even purchase a electronic device lock box. Make sure to use is for self monitoring and encourage your family to do the same, rather than using it for punishment.

- **Get an alarm clock:** Keep your phone away from your pillow by getting an alarm clock (preferably one without a snooze button). Make sleep a non-negotiable priority for both yourself and your family. Keeping phones away from the bedroom will help you instill mindful nighttime habits into your family's regular routine and replacing it with activities such as a relaxing bath, soft exercise, reading, or meditation.

- **Go screen-less for one night a week:** Pick a day of your choice every week to inform your friends, colleagues, and family members that you plan to go off the grid. Turn your phone on airplane mode and spend the night focusing on developing your relationship with your family, or doing something else that is important to you.

- **Make a conscious effort to partake in more non-technological activities:** Introduce activities that help you disconnect with the world, and the constant need to be (and feel) online all the time. Help your mind adjust to a mindset that is free of screen-related anxieties by fitting activities like walking, cooking, swimming, or making art into your family's routines.

- **Get friends and family to pitch in with their efforts and turn your digital detox into a group activity:** Setting challenges and comparing notes between yourselves can help motivate you to stick to your decisions and make your detox a fun way to connect with those around you. This activity can be done together or socially distanced, so get your mom friends together online, or distant family and challenge each other. Set reconvene times to discuss what worked and what didn't work after the challenge, and continue to take part in weekly or monthly challenges where you all choose certain days a week to digital detox.

Social Self-Care

Another form of caring for yourself is making sure that you are getting enough social interaction outside of your domestic circle. While your family may provide you with enough interaction to keep you from getting bored, switching social circles once in a while may be beneficial to you in several ways. Raising a child can often feel like fighting for an unseeable future, grounded by your personal connection to your child. Along with the joy that parenting surely brings, the degree of commitment required to raise a child will often result in isolating circumstances.

In short and in its most basic sense, making an effort to widen your circle could:

- help you feel heard, supported and not alone
- Provide you with a safe space to share your parenting concerns and discuss solutions with those who may have experienced similar concerns before you.
- allow you to connect with other people and widen your perspective on your approach toward life
- help you add a sense of order and control into your life where you are structuring something for you and not just your family.

On a personal level, connecting with friends (especially friends who also had kids) helped amp up my confidence and feel less alone in the endeavor of parenting. Connecting with people was a lot different from reading about their experiences through blogs. I appreciated both ways of learning about the scale of variety that people approach parenting with, but the former had a more grounding effect on me than the latter. Sharing real conversations with other mom friends, allowed me to appreciate how similar, yet vividly different the lives of several individuals within a community could be. One week I would be struggling to deal with my kid's fever and another's first experience with bullying, and the next I would manage to smile calmly as I informed my friends that things were okay. My life was colorful, unpredictable, and full of joy on its own when considering the beauty that children bring into the world; but adult conversation was an essential factor in helping me redefine the terms with which I had defined my life. As typical as it sounded, my children were the center of my universe, leaving me mostly satisfied with simply allowing myself to revolve around them like a loving (albeit tired) orbit. Being a mom means partially being immune to the call to let go, but a level of relaxation is a must in order to help yourself—and your children—grow as individuals. Regardless of the amount of research that you put into it, working solo never really amounts to the same amount of assurance, mixed opinions, and overall support that a group project can entail. I have found this to be true in parenting and in work and study. For parents with kids who do not necessarily conform to society's definitions of "good behavior," a few reassuring pats on the back go a long way.

Try working your way out of your parenting shell with these tips:

- **Make a habit of reaching out:** Do not wait for someone else to text you first. All of us are caught up in our own lives, but that doesn't mean that we *have* to be. There's nothing offensive about being reached out to. Let your ego slip to the back of your mind and be that one friend who bombards the group chat with funny memes. If calling feels like too much of an imposition, you can always text—or meme—your way back into rekindling a lost friendship. One of my closest friend relationships consists of only frequent memes back and forth on a weekly basis with a few words, and a monthly phone call to fill in the details and connect more deeply. Some people find it helpful to set a time schedule and a frequency to the number of times they reach out to people outside their domestic sphere. I like to maintain a casual schedule, but this works out to be roughly twice monthly. A more extroverted friend of mine typically spends each of her Fridays chilling with her girl squad—and while she doesn't have kids, many of her friends do and they show up because she schedules out the effort. Placing definitive expectations on your habits can help them manifest without becoming an added burden in your life, as you know that fulfilling these expectations, sets the course to be free of them. If you are more likely to thrive without order, hold onto the aspiration of working towards becoming more social in your mind as you navigate through your week.

- **Designate a weekly activity that you participate in with a group:** As we just touched on with Friday girls night, designating a weekly activity will provide you with a scheduled place and also a fixed time for you to connect with other people. A fitness-motivated group can help you multitask—you can use this time to connect emotionally and also look after yourself physically. Activities like pottery or knitting classes are other options that serve as both physical and mental self-care activities.

- **Find a support group:** Niche-interest support groups are very effective in helping people cater to specific social needs that may not be met by people in their immediate vicinity. A wealth of these groups exist online, but you can check for local groups as well since a touch of physical interaction always helps. As a parent new to sensory overload and seasonal eczema, online support groups acted almost exclusively as my support when no one else I knew closer had experience with these concerns themselves. My support group mothers were able to converse parenting with me in a way that left me feeling more lighthearted about where I believed I stood in life. My husband was supportive, but the connections I fostered through support groups—with women who had spent a similar amount of time researching early childhood-related sensory syndrome, providing me with the informed dialogue on the subject that was let's just say... more conversational and concerned than the degree of conversation I had with my husband which was usually along the lines of 'stop worrying, it's not that bad, it's all going to be fine'. I needed that too, but accompanied with a sense of shared worry only a mother knows.

- **Find and take advantage of your tribe:** As mentioned in previous chapters, your version of a girl gang can account for a quintessential level of change in your life. Maintain purposeful relationships with the women you value. Have meetups within, and without, the concept of child-rearing. Social contact will help you feel a lot less isolated, and it always helps to have several helping hands around you when you are raising a young child. I recently saw a group of influencer moms get together for a weekend away— without children in tow— and it elevated my spirit for how much we need our tribes. The fun, silliness, and connection to each other and themselves as individual identities outside of mothers was infectious! It made me want to hop through my phone and join them!

- **Surprisingly enough, having a pet can have a positive impact on you and your family:** Most parents often forego the prospect of owning a pet because they fear that they will be unable to manage the additional workload that comes with it. However, experts have found that tending to a pet has a mood-boosting effect on its caretakers. In making sure that your pet is fed, cleaned, and entertained, you are also taking a break from your own tasks to focus on a furry friend. Somewhat like child-rearing (but with far fewer expectations, pressure, and verbal rebuttals) cuddling your cat in the middle of the day can help balance stress-related cortisol levels in your body and increase its release of serotonin. Plus, your pet can also help build up your family's social skills—particularly by teaching them to be more empathetic and understanding of the needs of others. From a very young age, having a pet that needs to be looked after can provide your child with a basic understanding of how to look after others, essentially building on their more naturally egocentric perspective of the world.

Just as we have physical and mental needs, part of being human is being able to maintain coherent dialogue with the world around us. We need to feel and spread love, just as we need to recharge and work up a sweat, because—as productive as a 24-hour workday may be—it is impractical to push ourselves to structure our time on the sole basis of our obligations. Whether you are a stay-at-home mom, a working mom, or someone who straddles the line between the two, self-care is an essential part of sustaining your health. None of us can work around the clock for extended periods without feeling worn out. Furthermore, what such a work ethic promotes is only a chronic tendency to be weighed down by the burden that your tasks take upon you. Navigate the short days of mothering by prioritizing your help and comfort to significant levels. Remember, what you don't want to do is let these precious years of raising children, who are dependent on you both physically and emotionally, drift past you in your hurry to tackle your workload. You deserve to be happy and find joy in the life that you are leading. Your self-care is not a luxury. It is not something that has to be earned after a day of gruelling work. The sooner you realize this, the easier it will be for you to transition to a lifestyle that doesn't drain you of your energy.

CHAPTER 8

GET OUT OF YOUR HEAD

"You cannot have a positive life and a negative mind"
—JOYCE MEYER

Negative Mind, Negative Life

The number of times that you may have heard about the power of positive thinking may have been countless. Positivity is lauded for the way it is able to transform perspectives, relationships, and the lives they support. Health experts, fitness gurus, and motivational speakers swear by it. Personally, I remember considering this particular brand of positivity to be somewhat of a pipe dream. It seemed too simple of a solution—to simply make me feel better about my life issues. Looking back, I realize I was more afraid of looking stupid after making an informed attempt at changing the way I saw my life. If you are on the cusp of a breakthrough to change, you probably feel the same silliness with a glimmer of interest. Change puts you in a vulnerable place. I didn't want to position myself in a way that made me an easy target for judgment and criticism. However, it took a deeper look at negativity to teach me why positivity was able to provide such a tremendous level of change in so many lives.

The reason why opposing mindsets seem to create such polarized tendencies is because of the all-consuming nature that our mindsets have on how we see our lives. Consider a glass of water, and the famous saying about seeing it either half empty or half full. As cliché as the saying goes, our predisposition toward what we see plays a significant role in how we perceive it. We condition our bodies to think in certain ways and, once we do, we tend to stick to this bubble-like framework of thought, even outside its immediate context. On a scientific basis, you could think this is all an effect of how we are wired to exist. In order to protect ourselves from danger, we must stand vigilant against unforeseeable hostility. This translates to a sense of defensiveness as we commonly expect the worst out of things. A negative outlook toward the world around you may influence how you see all that is around you. Just as the ideological half-glass implies, negativity makes us dismissive of our own blessings, and results in a warped vision of the world. Health experts say that a tendency to lean toward negative overthinking can reinforce conditions like chronic stress, which may increase the likelihood of adverse health issues.

Part of the reason why a negative mindset is heavily advised against is because of the way it is able to subtly affect multiple elements of our lives and the way we choose to live them. A habit of seeing things negatively can result in a low sense of self-esteem and a reactionary quality of aspiring toward lower-level goals. If you viewed yourself to be hopelessly incapable, would you be more or less likely to aim for goals that you believe you have a chance of achieving? An individual prone to be pessimistic about life may underestimate their potential. When you doubt yourself to the level that you overthink every opportunity that comes your way, (which can also lead to sleepless nights and stress-related headaches), your capacity to succeed in life may be limited by your poor belief. What this results in is a topsy-turvy relationship between your self-esteem and the results that life seems to be throwing at you. In contrast, someone with a more positive impression of themselves will be more likely to apply to tasks considered to be beyond their conventional limits, leaving them with more chances at the lucky draw.

Take our example in relation to the confidence gap and how it affects men and women differently in the workplace. While it may seem silly to devote so much time and effort to something as intangible as building your sense of mindfulness, a lack of confident self-assessment has been connected to repercussions with very tangible, financially-worrying results. What a combination of mismatched Instagram posts, snippets of motivational speeches, and a dump of random positivity quotes unanimously beg of you is a change of perspective that will inadvertently save you from the cost of doubting yourself. While negative thinking may be an easy corner for you to bully yourself into, you don't deserve to suffer its consequences.

A few years back, my sister and I sporadically got matching tattoo's representing this when she was visiting me in Toronto. As children, we used to frequent a field behind our house that was covered in overgrown brush; particularly buttercups and dandelions. As we were walking through the tall grass one afternoon with our father, he turned to us and said 'Wow kids look at all the weeds' as white fluff drifted through the air potentially bringing on spring allergies that would lead to congested noses and weeping eyes. Being somewhere around the ages of four and six years, she and I looked at each other and closed our distance to earshot of each other to whisper *'No, look at all the wishes!'*

Whenever I'm feeling pessimistic, I think of this and remember—perspective is everything. We now have matching tattoo's of a dandelion papas —or wish— with our initials R and K around it. It's a wonderful reminder to me to always try and look on the bright side.

Overthinking and Its Effects on Motherhood

Overthinking isn't a clinical condition, but it's more of a time-consuming habit that gets the best of us quite frequently. Most commonly, overthinking causes us to spiral into ruminations about the past or anxieties about the future. Overthinking can also take the form of repetitive worries about the present—worrying about your perceived self-image or identity falls into this category. It presents itself as the what-if that keeps us up at night even when we are painstakingly tired. It comes to you in the dead of the night, as the centre of opportunity that always seems to drift past you when all else is quiet and resting. Overthinking is wondering if your life would look any different if you substitute its characters with other people, and it's places with new destinations. Overthinking can come to us in all different forms, but generally speaking, it's an unproductive, often circuitous form of thinking that stalls you rather than leading you anywhere worthwhile. The only place overthinking got me was in a google search at 2am, researching and certainly more confused and overwhelmed about my toddlers eating habits, and if he were getting enough or not sufficiently being nourished for his charted growth…which I was also tracking and over-thinking about.

As a mother, it is quite natural to be anxious about your little one and their well-being. Your overthinking may stem from an intrinsic self-defense mechanism, or come to be a habitual quality that you may resort to sticking to. It is unlikely that you push yourself to do this on purpose, but rather that your mind casually slinks into spiraling as an activity that it is conditioned to do. To some people, overthinking can be a conventional part of their thinking process—subtly taking up time and hindering their decision-making skills. To others, overthinking may be a warped form of the mind seeking to find comfort in the elimination of supposed risks—many women who suffer from postpartum anxiety may fall under this category, spending their waking moments with their young children stilled by the anxious fear of them being injured by some trick circumstance. I was that mother as much as I believe most of you are too. If you are not an over-thinker, take a moment to express gratitude to your centred mind.

As a bottom line, the helplessness that overthinking brings about may be rooted in genuine emotions of love or fear. But as with all aspects of our lives, practicing limits can help protect us from extremes that put ourselves and our families at risk. Someone with a habitual tendency to overthink will find the habit of overthinking to affect various elements of their lives and we should not pretend that sleep-related problems, and mental health issues like anxiety or depression are not dangerous to our well-beings. As a mother, facing the prospect of bringing up a child with the sheer force of will and instinct you had not used prior to birthing your child, it is important to keep an eye out for this kind of behavior.

If you experience any of the following signs, chances are that you may be a serial over-thinker:

- You have a tendency to relive shameful or embarrassing moments from your past in your head.
- Your mind keeps you up at night with how it spirals in uncontrollable worrying thoughts.
- You think deeply about the maybes and what-ifs of your life frequently.
- You have a tendency of replaying conversations that you had with people in your head, often attempting to read between the lines to look for a secret meaning. This may lead to mulling over what you could have said or done differently in response.
- You have a habit of tormenting yourself with the memory of what you believe to be your mistakes— this is my worst.
- On the occasion that someone speaks or acts in a way that bothers you, you tend to spend a large amount of time thinking about their behavior.
- Sometimes your thoughts lead you to be oblivious of things happening around you, removing yourself mentally from present situations.

- You have a tendency to worry about things that you have no control over. These worries burden you and make it difficult for you to focus on whatever you are doing.
- You tend to run through worst-case scenarios before taking any course of action. I am also super guilty of this one.

The tricky part about all of this lingers in the fact that during the process of problem-solving, there lies a fine line between overthinking and critical thinking. Quite easily, you can be under the impression that you are working on finding solutions to your worries when your thoughts actually hinder your progress toward productive goals. The anxiety or depression that an overthinking habit can bring on has physical repercussions such as fatigue, headaches, and a loss of appetite. Over long periods of time, overthinking can affect your way of life quite significantly by negatively affecting the way in which you perceive the world around you.

Modern-day moms become inevitably afflicted by overthinking, as our appetite for the information that we seek about raising our children overloads us. From the moment our children are born, we are given decisions and choices between various opinions that all seem to have an effect on their long-term development. I remember making my first anxiety-filled parenting choice when I was taught how to hold my son for the first time in the hospital. The paediatrician showed me a few way to support his neck while I cradled him or picked him up. I remember the picture of an infographic showing how if he lay on his back too long, his head would flatten. On one hand, lying down would be more comfortable, given the new scar on my abdomen that was still fresh and raw from surgery. On the other, I wanted to do what was best by picking him up and holding him and showing him that I was his ever-capable mama. This is where overthinking, and inevitable anxiety seeps in. The fact that I was worried, meant I was doing just fine. Then it was the first nights sleep at home that brought on intense anxiety over SIDS. The anxieties worked like the steady pace of attempting to walk up a reverse escalator. Each step of progress I made was met with a new step to worry about, and I still never got ahead. These concerns that fed my overthinking told me that I had to be actively in a state of stress, all the time.

We all want to do what's best for our children, but have no way of proving our efforts. What's left from this equation is the difficult job of constantly having to assess ourselves, through both flawed lenses of our own and those of society. Our situation is like trying to avoid mom burnout by sticking to disposable diapers instead of reusables, and then worrying about how we're going to make up for our carbon footprint, or the additional garbage tags we need to pick up and pay for, and remember to put on our bin to be picked up on garbage day because we are producing more than the city limits of waste since we had a baby human in the house peeing and pooping 7 times a day.

In spite of how vast our decisions seem (and how foresighted our anxiety makes us feel), certain outcomes will always be out of our control. Worrying about your decision to have not sent your kid to playgroup or pre-k and how that connects to their speed of acquiring language may be rich food for thought, yet unproductively so—only resulting in you being burdened with an unnecessary and unproductive thinking session.

Let's dive into what you can do about it!

Understand Your Thought Patterns

One of the key factors that influence how we perceive the world around us is how our minds are predisposed to process these perceptions. Experts call these factors cognitive distortions, which are patterns of thinking that act as filters (or biases) that influence how we are programmed to receive situations that affect us. In simple terms, your mind may be wired—by bad mental habits and negative environmental influences—to think of certain things in a particular way. Think of these as prejudices that your mind may hold against you that are able to turn situations into worse versions of themselves. However, being prejudiced to think negatively does not mean that you will be doomed to a life of pessimism. A conscious effort to be more mindful of your mental behavior and tendencies can help you manifest the positivity you put into practice. All this takes is patience, consistency, and a bit of self-awareness.

Cognitive distortions may come to you in a variety of shapes and forms. In the following section, I will list and describe the most common ones, which mothers are considered to revel in.

Personalization

This term can be attributed to behavioral biases that assume personal faults as default, regardless of the other factors that affect the situation. For example—your son doesn't eat his lunch and it's because you are not doing good enough as a mother, or your daughter has a tendency to need you by her side at night (and you feel like this is because you didn't enforce enough independent activities during the COVID-19 lockdown period when she had been fresh out of the womb and you feared for the future. Or, for instance, someone says something harsh to you, and it's either because you do not assert yourself enough or you just let them push you around.

A nature that makes you inclined to reserve blame for yourself as an internal default can be understood as personalization. Of course, this can lead to situations where you perceive the world in a way that is entirely untrue. What the reality may look like is, your son may not have had a good appetite that day (because he was fresh out of his seasonal flu, and may have needed some time to work his palate), or your daughter may be meant to hit the independent sleeping milestone a bit later than the other children you compare her to. Neither of these are your faults. That friend who said something awful to you may have been having a bad day at work, which caused them to unfairly project their negative emotions onto you.

Remember, not everyone has others' best interests in mind, and not everyone lives up to the appearance of normalcy that they hold toward you. What personalization has the capacity to do with it's distorted perception, is gaslight your understanding of reality so that you are unfairly to blame in uncomfortable situations. Certain things exist out of our control and attributing blame to ourselves will not change them—it will only succeed in making us feel worse about ourselves without any productive reason to do so.

Mind Reading

Mind reading occurs when we interpret the behavior of others and use our personal interpretations as a basis for critical judgment. While an ability to interpret the words and behavior of other people may be beneficial to you in certain circumstances, a habitual quality of doing this may lead you to forget about how subjective interpretation is.

For instance, assuming that a partner doesn't do their part of the chores because you *think* they consider it beneath them to do so, is an example of mental distortion at play. Without apparent facts proving what you believe, your mind is under the impression that what it is biased toward believing can substitute for the truth. However, the only person who can interpret your partner's speech and actions is them. You have no way of truly deciphering thoughts, no matter how close you may be to them. Maybe you have more to communicate about the division of labor in the household and the way it weights on you. Maybe your partner finds themselves to be incompetent at certain aspects of household work you wish them to assist in if you have high standards. You can never truly know unless proven otherwise, which is why it is so important that you become aware of the cognitive distortions that you may be accustomed to following. Never assuming and opening up the conversation in a non assumptive way can drastically change the outcome of a situation that is irritating you.

Magnifying

Magnifications are cognitive distortions that make little things amount to a greater significance than they actually possess. As we navigate the experience of living, even without factoring the added element of young children into the equation, we will find that it is hard to tame life into the neat lines of our careful plans. Mishaps happen and bodies get tired—and in spite of how cautious we are, it is rare that everything will always go exactly to plan. With children, the level of unpredictability that our lives seem to hold multiplies tenfold. In their fascinating journey toward growth, it is hardly likely that they can grasp the expectations that we have for them. A tendency to magnify "issues" that we see in life will lead us to have a false negative perception of the way we live, and it could be a trait our children eventually learn from us.

For instance, your toddler has a potty-related accident. Either he went in his pants, or he did something to make the situation ickier than the way you had trained him to. You had spent the last four months patiently training him out of his diapers and this accident, one among many, seems to have the power to break you. It doesn't have to, though. You can still have a good day, even if you had to clean him up —and possibly other surfaces. If you allow your mind to magnify the significance of a single mishap to overwhelm the capacity of an otherwise peaceful, fun and enjoyable day, you will have several more bad days to face than ever truly cast on you. The key factor in processing something unexpected is deciding how far you will allow it to affect you. In raising children and sustaining relationships with your loved ones, it is important that you do not allow the negatives to overwhelm the positives, as this frame of thought will likely blind you to the possible positives that life could bring your way. If you have ever been blessed with rain on your wedding day, then you know exactly what I'm talking about.

Catastrophizing

People catastrophize when they assume the worst, making a mountain out of a molehill. A bit similar to magnifying (yet with the element of imagining outcomes that tend to add to the sense of worry that the situation is attributed to), catastrophizing is a cognitive distortion that is capable of shaping individually innocent events into potentially catastrophic circumstances. You catastrophize when you assume that your husband showing up half an hour late from work is proof of an affair and his disinterest in you. You catastrophize when you push yourself to believe that every bout of childhood sickness is going to lead to your kid being hospitalized with a rare child-related disease.

Yes, some aspects of our lives are beyond our control. Yet, making a habit of imagining every possible reason for individual elements of your life will lead you to a path of being unable to find any source of joy or gratitude in it. Take what you know, even if you don't feel like you can trust it, and place significance on fact rather than personal interpretations—because it's at this stage that your mind's mental prejudices can distort the meaning that you are programmed to perceive. You cannot predict what you will eventually have to experience. Even if you dread these surprises, find comfort in the sense of normality that you experience on a daily basis, and work yourself up from there. A habit of assuming the worst will only instill fear of life in general, so accepting this form of cognitive distortion has the potential to have significant ripple effect for your mind where you worry less, and get back to living more.

Emotional Reasoning

Emotions are powerful, as they are abstract. Emotional reasoning occurs when we decide to take what we feel about something to be a reality. While our emotions do serve a purpose, and it is helpful to try and figure out why we feel certain ways about certain events, an over-reliance on emotive reasoning can result in feelings of intense anxiety. This happens because, as sure as we are about how we feel about things, our emotions represent an exaggerated response to reality. Sometimes our first reactionary response toward an event may not be faithful toward the real world in its absoluteness. This makes the actions that we take based on our emotional reasoning highly uncertain. For instance, on a day when you are slightly off your normal routine—maybe you slept past your alarm clock and made up for lost time by tossing your kid a granola bar or ego waffles as you run out the door—your emotional reasoning for a perceived failing of yours might not be representative of reality, in the actual sense of the word. Your internalized anger for straying off the course of your ideal routine may leave you feeling guilty for not making a more organic meal that will keep them full for more of the day. This guilt could build into the emotional reasoning that you are irresponsible, shaping a chain of further behavioral tendencies, which may cause you to go back and forth between attesting to and rebelling against the emotional reasoning that you have associated with yourself.

Having experienced this myself, I often translated my poor emotional reasoning to a push and pull between setting underwhelming expectations for myself and pushing myself to meet expectations that were beyond my capacity of always fulfilling. I would end up doing things like boil the water with much content for a 'lazy' Mac and cheese dinner (that the kids were fine with) before quickly changing my mind and putting the pot back into the cupboard so that I could clean the counter for an endeavor of making pizza dough from scratch. Meanwhile, an objective survey of my family's daily food intake compared to nutritious food groups —that I usually made a point of serving—would tell me that I was right on track to where a family with young kids could aspire to be... if not better.

However, even if rational reasoning proves us wrong, the bias that our minds are conditioned to practice will only enforce a negative self-image for us. Similarly, if your mind emotionally reasons that you are overweight, you have an increased chance of conceding to this assumption—even if your bodily statistics prove you to be in a healthy weight range. In this manner, cognitive distortions can warp our understanding of our reality to be one which dissatisfies and disappoints us, leaving us helpless to the awful force of pent-up emotions.

Blaming

Blaming is an anti-responsibility distortion and one that I now cringe at the most. If an individual has a predisposition against taking responsibility, they tend to deflect blame toward another person. This causes the formation of undue accusations, and behavior that targets other individuals unnecessarily. What may seem like a minor flaw in being unable to admit blame out loud, leads to misdirected hate. This kind of behavior will take many forms. For instance—you've woken up late, and you don't have enough time to prepare for your weekend trip that you planned a week earlier. Your partner gets agitated for running behind because the traffic will be worse. He has already gotten ready on time and has fed and dressed the kids. You discussed the night before that you would pack lunches in the morning so that they were fresh. You decide to place blame on your partner for not forcing you out of bed when he gently nudged you a few times with a friendly reminder because he felt bad being too pushy. You blame your toddler for not waking you up like a feral animal like he always does on weekends... just not this one. What this distortion will eventually lead to is impending problems with no viable solutions left in sight, as rightful blame has been deflected.

By this example, blaming your husband or toddler for your own slip-up will do little to help you get ready on time—this will only amount to a succession of days where you fail to correct yourself by waking up at the correct time and misappropriate blame because you have placed the responsibility of correction on someone else. If practiced frequently, your mind will habitually blame instead of focusing on your own self-growth, potentially becoming a cause of stunted relationships and hindered personal development. Own your faults, lead by example, and take responsibility to minimize the snowball effect of assigning blame for your mistakes to others. Owning your own accountability will exemplifying the importance and the expectation for others in your household to do the same.

Filtering

Filtering distorts your perspective of life in a way that focuses on the negative, and then dismisses the positives entirely. This cognitive distortion warps your understanding of reality in a way that makes it emphatically pessimistic. Comparable to someone who is only able to see a bad grade on a report card (instantly forgetting all the positive achievements around it), mental filtering can create a polarized version of reality that illegitimates the optimistic parts of your life. An individual used to this frame of mind will likely rule out the positives in their life, attributing them to luck, while consciously believing that the negative aspects of their lives can be owed to their inherent nature and predispositions as individuals. A mind conditioned toward this form of thinking may leave you vulnerable to numerous depressive disorders, due to its nature of circumventing your experience of reality in a way that overtly pushes you toward negativity over the positive aspects of your life.

Perfectionism

Perfectionism is a mental bias that causes you to hold yourself to impossible standards that are incredibly difficult to meet. This could lead to you seeing all and every kind of achievement to be a disappointment in contrast to your unreachable standards, setting the pace for a vicious cycle of toxic overwork. Remember, these biases are not exclusively individualistic. They affect the lives of our loved ones as intensely (possibly even more) than they affect our own, which is why it is important that we practice awareness of our own mental habits.

If you are inherently used to comparing everything that you see to impossible standards, it may be difficult for you to appreciate what your loved ones achieve in life. For example, if you are too busy comparing your husbands acts of love to grander gestures that you envision for yourself in your head, you will find it tough to be thankful for the effort that they *do* put forward in their own right. Im not dismissing that our husbands should sometimes put in a bit more of an effort, but have you stopped to think about any small things that they have been doing for you? You may find it difficult to enjoy life when you measure yourself by an unreachable ideal of a Hallmark holiday special. Constantly disappointed at your inability to reach your impossible standards? Your mind will be biased against appreciating your actual achievements, depriving you of the potential joy that you could have otherwise sought from them. What results is a constant feeling of being underwhelmed when reality fails to live up to ideological perfection.

Polarizing

Polarizing is when your mind automatically assumes an all-0r-nothing perception of the people and events in your lifetime. This kind of belief jumps to extremities, leaving subjects either entirely "bad" or "good." Many of their thoughts may be filled with words like "all," "none," "never," and "always." These words affirm a solid stance toward the opinion considered, leaving little room for flexibility. An individual with this form of cognitive distortion will have a hard time coming to terms with occasions that are not entirely good, but not bad either—or the other way around. They will also have a hard time reconciling experiences that shelter both sides of the coin, leaving experiences with mixed emotions to be misappropriated into staunch categories of black and white. A perspective of this nature holds harsh repercussions for the prospect of motherhood, where the unpredictable behavior of growing children often accounts for several highs and lows, and rarely a definite "goodness" or "badness." It can be hard for people conditioned toward this form of thinking to embrace the joy of motherhood, or admit the likelihood of burnout when they feel fulfilled with the role they play for their families. This can lead to the overwhelming extremes of either black or white, resulting in several drawbacks as we live in a world that operates in shades of grey and variance of color. Trying to cram perceptions into only one of two categories can blur the lines between right and wrong.

The 'Should Have'

A person with a *should have* mental behavioral habit for their day (or week) falls into the trap of constantly reassessing and being critical of a past that is no longer under their control. The *should have* person has a high chance of spending a long time ruminating about the consequences of their actions and how they 'should have' acted in a better, or more appropriate way, leaving them to dwell in the past. Does this sound like you? While practicing self-awareness may be a commendable habit, it's hardly likely that you use your self-criticism as a basis for self-growth, and instead choose to use it as a platform to shame yourself for not holding up to impossible standards of perfection. It can also lead you to dealing with mental blocks for fairly trivial matters that do not mean as much to other people as they do to you.

Consider this—your partner leaves for work in a hurry, forgetting to say goodbye and giving you a quick kiss as they usually do when they rush toward the door with a coffee and bagel in hand. You could spend the entire day going over your own behavior, torturing yourself about which conditional alternatives could have changed the behavior and that missed kiss you desired. In reality, the missed action had nothing to do with you at all, and he was just running late and was thinking about a presentation that day. The egocentric nature of most of these cognitive distortions often saturate reality to be directly relational to your actions and attitudes as a person, when the truth is that the world proves to be far more sophisticated than our simplistic self-loathing thoughts.

Of course, we aren't to be blamed for the nature of our thoughts. Our childhood and upbringing could have conditioned us to owe accountability for actions that are beyond our control. The quickest way to avoid dialogue about a complex issue is to blame one side. Often, we take this blame upon ourselves or attribute it entirely to our loved ones or circumstances. However, much of the human experience is dialogic in nature. Wiping out a single side of the bushfire is hardly likely to tame its fiery blaze, as it runs rampant. Self-awareness of the cognitive distortions and increased tendencies that we have toward these things, will help direct us to having a better understanding of our lives, and the events that surround them. A key step toward this change is redefining our relationship with our minds, allowing ourselves due agency over our own mental habits.

So what could you have done about that missed kiss? Communicate in a self aware, non-blameful way. A quick kind text saying 'missed your kiss this morning honey. You are gonna smash this presentation out of the water— you got this!' Acknowledges the action but also puts consideration on the possible distraction, and a recognition of understanding for acceptance. The likelihood of you getting the response that puts your mind at ease, is much higher than if you left it to him, or if you said something like—'why didn't you say goodbye this morning?'.

Change Your Thinking

At this point, it is easy to feel helpless in the face of the apparent power that cognitive distortions can possibly hold over you. Chin up—all is not lost. Cognitive distortions may seem scary on paper, though they are actually part of the toxic thought patterns that we engage with on a daily basis. As overwhelming as it is to deal with the promise of something that your mind has naturally been conditioned toward doing, with enough practice and awareness, these distortions can be studied and redefined so that they don't affect you as much. Let's evaluate.

Cognitive restructuring is a technique that works at the root of cognitive behavioral therapy (CBT). It operates by analyzing and assessing distortions in accordance with their triggers and effects, and the objective oversight of their rationality. When you restructure your negative thoughts, you reframe them in a way that is less irrational and easier to deal with. Doing so will help you expand your perspective of yourself, your capabilities as an individual, and your view of the world around you. If you have had the privilege to travel the world, it can feel similar to that moment you realize how diverse the world is, and how insignificant your problems are to the bigger picture. Getting on a plane and seeing the city or town you live in as a small dot beneath the clouds truly pulls you out of your narrow perspective. We have the ability to do this with our minds internally. Like all tasks that require you to reverse a particular change, you will have to trace your way back to the root causes of your negative feelings in a manner that is systematic, breaking down complexities to their simplest forms. Lean into your senses of touch, taste, smells and sounds. Recognize the roots and write down your possible triggers and reactions.Reframing your negative thought patterns will help you practice more kindness and positivity, allowing you to grow into a version of yourself that will be less vulnerable to toxic self-blaming. It may not change overnight, but with time and practise, you can significantly alter your tendencies towards negative thought patterns and find greater peace for yourself in the present moments.

Check In With Yourself

One of the first steps that you can take to successfully reframe your thinking pattern is to increase the sense of awareness that you have of yourself. Make a habit of noticing your feelings. In the beginning, you might find it difficult to do so, because your cognitive biases might seem like they come naturally to you. Separating the warped reality (which you see as a result of the cognitive distortions that you might hold within you) from an objective version of your experience may come as a tough job. Still, it is not an impossible task. Keeping a journal, or any other form of a mood log, can be a helpful way for you to become more aware of your emotional state of mind. On the occasion that you feel like you are overwhelmed, check in with yourself.

Ask yourself the following questions:

- Am I focusing on the work at hand?
- Do I feel disconnected from my current reality?
- Does my body show physical signs of being overwhelmed (increased heart rate or a feeling of dizziness)?
- When did I begin to experience these signs? Were they triggered by a particular occurrence?

Once you've got a clear idea of how you register an emotional outburst, you will find it easier to get ahead of your mind in its practice of pushing thoughts toward a negative narrative. Ask yourself these questions each time you feel overwhelm engulfing you, and you will find it easier to control and manage your emotions.

Identify Your Negative Thoughts

What are your worst thoughts? What kind of thoughts tend to linger with you, long past when they started, sending you down obsessive spirals that drain you of your energy? Once you've checked in on yourself, make a habit of getting down to the specifics. Try not to label your feelings too abstractly. For instance, consider that you feel overwhelmed at the changing room of a popular clothing store. Making the connection between your negative emotions and the specific insecurities that you have with regards to your body image can help you make sense of your stressed state of mind. The more you know about your thoughts, the easier it will be for you to hunt the triggers that cause you to think them. The 360° florescent lit room of mirrors was without a doubt a trigger for my negative thoughts on my post baby body. Taking the time to identify how stress (or a sense of being overwhelmed) makes you feel may aid you in finding ways to cope—therefore, being a necessary skill for learning how to manage your emotions. Unless I am feeling particularly brave, I opt for trying on clothes at home.

A simple way to help you identify your thoughts is to subject them to a critical assessment, you can use this technique:

1. When you feel something negative about yourself, write the thought down. Do not extrapolate on this. Do not attempt to reason with the thought, or justify its rationality. You might be too overwhelmed to deal with it objectively, so take it in stride.
2. Connect this thought to a specific location, or event. Hone in on details like how frequently you catch yourself thinking this thought—or thoughts of a similar nature—and note them down as well.
3. Now that you've arrived at your thought, and associated it with a particular event, consider how it makes you feel. Be careful to be specific about your emotions. If you are having a hard

time articulating the emption, look at a feelings wheel/ wheel of emotion.
4. Make an assessment of these thoughts on a weekly basis. Group together thoughts of a similar nature. Narrow down thoughts that leave you feeling particularly distressed—you might find it beneficial to flag these down for you to address at a later date.

Identifying your thoughts will help you associate them with specificity, rather than leaving them to be indefinite in their abstractness. Making a habit of noting down your thoughts will help you instill meaning and order to the vast rush of emotion that you deal with on a daily basis.

Question Assumptions

As you revisit your notes from the above technique, subject them to a close analysis. *Do not* allow yourself to accept any of your thoughts as absolute truths.

Taking care to read each of your notes carefully, ask yourself the following questions:

- Is this particular thought supported by facts, or is it more based on emotion? In other words, is your thought a fact or an opinion?
- Is there any kind of proof supporting this thought?
- Can this thought be validated? Which proportion of your thought seems accurate and which proportion of your thought can be discredited?
- Can this thought be proved by any form of testing or evaluation?
- If this thought is true, at its most earnest, how would this affect you? Does the potential credibility of this thought harm you in any way that is worth the distress it brings you?
- Can the context with which you processed your thought be used to interpret it in any other way?

In spite of how strongly you feel about a certain idea or situation, an assumption without proper and accurate evidence fails to be anything greater than what it is—a strongly felt assumption. Most of the time, we allow the power of our emotions to overcome our better reasoning. Questioning your assumptions can be an efficient way in which you can let rationality take charge of the narrative that you want your mind to follow.

Evaluate Evidence

When a negative thought comes your way, subject it to a critical evaluation. Your mind is a temple, and you need to protect it from unnecessary and intrusive thoughts. The moment you start to spot the telltale signs of anxiety, note down your thoughts. Tell yourself that you can either choose to believe this thought or disregard it entirely if it is in fact just you being hard on yourself. On a plain sheet of paper, draw a line straight down the middle. On the left side of the page, write down the evidence that you have for this thought. On the right side, write down the evidence you have against this thought. Remember to be objective. You don't always have to bat against yourself. Let's say you've just thought of yourself as a bad parent. You've written down your cave in for unhealthy cereal choices and *Cocomelon* habits as your single most disgraceful motherly practices. Yes there could be some room for improvements here... but remember the why. The endless sacrifices that you've made since the birth of your child; the nights of no sleep leading to one less fought battle in the morning or fever fests that required entertainment of the TV more than usual. These considerations can make your first list seem a bit silly, in hindsight. Do not attempt at discrediting, or at disqualifying, any aspects of either of your lists because of how much they contrast with each other, this is simply an evaluative process.

Thoughts grow to become scary and overwhelming when we let them hover over us, like ghosts that we are too afraid to confront. Once transferred to a different medium (like an unassuming piece of paper), many of these thoughts lose their power over us, as your mind may have unwittingly been provoked to read them objectively in the absence of the fear that you first associated them with. Part of why this exercise is so effective is because it makes use of what you already know in order to put things into perspective. So, let your thoughts flow without the fear of holding them back. When you are done, look over your page and make an informed choice about which thoughts you want to believe.

Avoid Generalizing

Once you've established a habit of seeing everything in an all-or-nothing manner, you've likely built a practice of using your most negative thoughts to make a generalization of your mood—often overriding many positives with the few negatives that you cannot seem to shake off. You may generalize when your toddler wets the bed once, and take this as proof of how they will *never* learn to control their bladders in the night. You may generalize when you stub your toe and take on the rest of your entire day pessimistically. When we generalize, we let our vision of the world blur over the good details in our need to zoom in on the bad.

A great way to counter a habit of generalizing is to subject your thoughts to a game of opposites. For instance, if you are feeling like you will never be good at your job, think of three factors about your work habits—such as your punctuality, work ethic, and determination—that prove otherwise. The most important part about this exercise is teaching yourself that life doesn't work in all-consuming ways, even when it is able to cause all-consuming pain. Cognitive restructuring works by helping you shape the way you register emotions. Your emotions may still come to you unpredictably, hitting you at full force with their impact, but the benefit of cognitive reframing lies in how your mind learns to look out for the debris and proactively brace itself from the particular hit that it is conditioned to receive. You are training yourself to read the language of your emotions, instead of simply taking the brunt of the hits that life throws at you. Generalizing is a sneaky mindset that can creep up on us more when we are sleep deprived, so be conscious of how many hours of sleep you have had prior to finding yourself in a generalizing mindset. Understand that if you have been running on nothing, it is not you— an engine can't run efficiently if it's sputtering on it's last drop of gas.

Replace Shoulds

Many of the people who I have had the pleasure of meeting in my life— friends, family, and myself included—experience living to be tough. Life is not easy for most people. Most of us are never pleased enough with how we exist—which is all right, considering how we all have our goals and aspirations that we would like to work toward. However, the race toward productivity—the clean room, the color-coded wardrobe, the aesthetically pleasing day planner—leaves most of us too exhausted to ever consider the concept of committing to other endeavors willingly. It is always something we dread—the work that we *have* to do.

Experts say that it is the inflexibility of *having* to do something, rather than simply doing it by choice, that makes compulsory acts seem so difficult to accomplish. You should not have to *should* anything in your life. There are no rules. While goals are one of the best ways to kick-start your work productively, it is important that you keep them from taking the joy away from your labor. Take control of your aspirations, and add an element of choice to them. Replace the *shoulds* and *musts* of your goals with a more flexible language. We do this with our kids all the time, so why not with ourselves?

For instance, if you plan on reading more books this year, change your aspiration from, "I should be reading 10 books this year," to, "I can read up to 10 books this year." The former example is more rigid and result-driven than the latter. While a firm mentality *may* be beneficial in helping you achieve your goals, it is important that you see to your mental welfare in your drive toward productivity. Say it out loud. Do you hear the subtle difference? How does each statement make you feel? Our lives constantly provide us with trade-offs between our well-being and various other aspects of our lives. Taking care to protect our sense of wellness can help preserve our motivation for work of greater quality than that which our exhausted minds are able to conjure. Saying 'I can' rather than 'I should' ignites the excitement of optimism for the task at hand. It sends our brains an internal spark of confidence for something that we want to do and not just something that we should be doing.

Generate Alternatives

By now, it must have grown seemingly evident how subtly your mental distortions can disguise themselves to be the truths that you live by. For you to move on from the roadblocks that your mind pushes your way, you need to forge alternate routes that you can dodge them with. One of the key concepts of cognitive reframing is widening the narrowed perspective caused by pessimistic emotions. You need to explore alternatives. Some of them can act as counters to your negative thoughts. Instead of feeling like '*I am unappealing to others, or my body is not flattering this dress today*', you can repeat positive affirmations such as, '*I am happy with the way I look in these jeans*' instead, as a determined way to move past the kind of thinking that you have grown accustomed to.

Other alternatives can come to you as solutions to the roadblocks that your brain keeps placing in your way. Many of us mothers yearn to learn something new after we have children, we cast the net out for a newfound identity. If you always find a certain subjects that you wished you were better in way too hard, some helpful alternatives would be getting a tutor to help you or practicing different learning habits to help you understand the subject better. You can also generate alternatives in the way you choose to *react* to certain situations. For instance, if you feel like your coworkers or judgemental teachers at your child school treat you poorly or make negative assumptions about you, you can channel the internal conventional self-loathing into making sure that you will appear confident and unaffected by them. This is an important first step to actually not caring. The appearance of confidence can have profound effect on your true self confidence. The importance of generating alternatives is that you prove to yourself how vast your options are, widening your view of the world from the skewed perspective that your mind has been warped into believing. There is no one perspective on the world, not for you, not for anyone— so let that potential pitfall go before you fall too deep into it!

Practice Compassion

As a final note, the most powerful way that you can reclaim control over your emotions is by forcing yourself to practice compassion. Many of the mental distortions that work within us cause us to be biased against ourselves. They make us discredit our achievements, disqualify sources of joy, and have a tendency of draining us of the positive energy that we could have otherwise spent on ourselves. *You deserve kindness.*

In the most rudimentary sense of the concept, you deserve kindness as you are every ounce of the human being that you are able to see in other people. We often fall into the habit of accommodating the emotions and needs of the people around us, without regarding our own sense of mental stability and emotional wellness. Reverse this form of thought and work toward lessening the pressure that the world tends to put on your shoulders. Tell yourself you are exactly where you need to be for this moment. Allow yourself the little mishaps and accidents that you allow for other people in your life. Recognize your challenges and appreciate the effort that you have been making to exist, kindly and compassionately, in a world that has proved to be very cruel to caregivers. By making an effort to surround yourself with positive thoughts, you will find it less stressful and intimidating to attempt your inner goals even if nothing else has changed.

Not So Hypothetical: Questions to Ask Yourself

- What cognitive distortions do you feel you practice most frequently against yourself?
- Why do you think these distortions affect you in the way that they do?
- How would you approach reframing the mental biases that you consider to hold you back?

CHAPTER 9

CREATING YOUR MOM-IFESTO

> Permission to move forward with boldness
> is never given by the fearful masses
> —BRENDON BURCHARD

The What and Why of a Personal Manifesto

I became obsessed with manifesto's during my University years, when I was introduced to them in a cultural revolutions class. I wrote down many for myself involving my desire to self-grow, land the career I wanted, and much more. A personal manifesto serves to be a declaration of what you want from your life. It will entail how you treat different circumstances that life will throw your way, using your core values as a basis through which you will measure the way you approach the world. At first glance, this may seem a bit strange. Most of us simply want to carry on with our lives without much drama, and a personal manifesto may seems like a pointless way of putting things into perspective. Many of the influencing figures and news providers we follow today would associate the concept of a personal manifesto with supervillains and serial killers, to my utter exasperation. What most see in the concept of commandeering their vision for their life on paper, is either an eccentric perspective of life or a twisted version of it. Still, I insist that normal people have just as much force in their life as the next Marvel supervillain to push into a personal manifesto.

We are all the sum of our experiences, upbringings, and the change that these factors provoke us into wanting from the world. Think of a personal manifesto as a quick way of illustrating the person you want to be for yourself on paper, using it as a mode through which you can motivate yourself to pursue your goals. Think of it as your "ultimate bucket list" that you will use to mold the best version of yourself. You approach various aspects of your life, which you otherwise experienced without much fanfare, and connect them with a purpose that you must fulfill in order to adhere to your manifesto. In pushing for this, I am not saying that your manifesto has to be a 100-page document that you will revisit every blue moon. Like a personal mantra, a manifesto can be a short and effective way of allowing yourself to reflect on your core values and work your way toward them. Even the most down-to-earth individuals, have their core ideals. The companies we lead and work for do too! A manifesto can help them assess their current realities in accordance to the innermost ideals that they set for themselves, using these ideals as a basis through which they can figure out how much work they need to be putting into their lives and business to make their goals a reality.

Your *mom-ifesto* can either be a vision of the ideal person you wish to be—removed from your motherhood—or a mix between your mom goals and your personal aspirations. The choice of your subject matter lies in your definition of motherhood and also your aspirations for yourself. It is not the presence or absence of the subject of motherhood that defines your mom-ifesto. A personal manifesto is a love letter to the individual that you hope to become in the future. Sure, motherhood is one of the nonreversible changes in our lives that we cannot imagine our futures without. However, it is important that you comprehend your life with a sense of individualism, choosing your goals and aspirations to suit your own needs rather than *going with the flow* in order to accommodate your loved ones. The choices you make in your own life, regardless of their association with your motherhood, have to possess a degree of intentionality. In writing a mom-ifesto, you are intending changes in your life for yourself, in the hopes that your will empowers you to take the actions necessary in order to bring them into existence.

Write a Personal Mom-ifesto

Pick the Topics

What you make of your mothering manifesto or 'mom-ifesto' is a choice of your own. It can be as personal, or as abstract, as you want to be—just as long as you keep in mind to be true to yourself and represent your desires most faithfully on paper. A ripped page from a lined notebook or the fanciest letterhead you have will do just fine if you want to make it feel official. Begin to write down the topics of your manifesto with something simple such as, "when in doubt." You could also go for options like, "dealing with pain," or, "how you should treat yourself." Think of specifics as you go on. The most difficult part is taking that first step and starting, so remember not to think too hard and to simply concentrate on putting the pen to paper.

A generic list of topics that you could approach for your mom-ifesto is:

- how you plan to approach your career
- your relationship with your spouse
- the way you intend to live
- your approach to parenting
- your ethics for life
- your carbon footprint
- how you plan to deal with tough decisions

- how you plan to deal with conflicts.

Use Visualization

Visualization is a core technique used by high performers to help them motivate themselves to achieve their goals. When you visualize, you imagine yourself experiencing the goals that you want to manifest in your life. The image of your success, in this context, acts as a key motivating factor for accomplishing your goals. Think of each of the topics you have picked out for your manifesto and consider how you want to deal with them.

For example, consider how you want to treat your mind. Do you want to be the kind of person who pressures yourself into accomplishing their goals, or do you want to approach yourself more compassionately? There is no right or wrong answer here, it is what works best for you. Think of what you assume to be the peak of mental self-care. This could be anything—from a fulfilling hobby to a scheduled hour of the day that you delegate to yourself. Envision yourself experiencing this goal. Imagine yourself spending an hour of your day strumming the guitar like no one's watching. Imagine yourself in your coziest sweater, curling up with your favorite book. Imagine yourself closing your work document and shutting down your laptop, casually moving to seat yourself by the television without guilt or shame, just doing it as something typical. Now, think of how this reality will make you feel— A moment of fun, a moment of peace, a moment of rest. Think of the feelings of innermost satisfaction and pride that achieving your goals might fill you with. Consider how this imagined change in your life will affect your loved ones. Personally, better mental self-care means that I can build a more comprehensive relationship with my husband, and be more patient with my children. Be very specific with your visualization for yourself. Remember, no one is watching you, so let loose of your inhibitions.

What you want to do is to encourage your unconscious mind to work toward your goals. Oddly similar to envying an influencer for their luxurious lifestyle (but without the toxic resentment), you can use your visual image of yourself to stir up the innermost desires that you seek. However, it is important that you do not use your visualization as a form of belittling or competing with yourself. Instead, convince yourself that you are seeing a vision of you from a linear future, and that your advancement will bring you closer to experiencing your reality soon enough. Visualization can help you hone in on the goals that you desire for yourself, and work toward bringing them into reality. They are not as far away as you think.

Analyze Your Current Situation

Take reality into account—do not diminish it, and do not shame yourself for it. Simply assess your current situation, working out the logistics of how much you will have to work to make your dreams an achievable reality. At this point, you need to make yourself aware of the gap between your life and the life you desire. It is important that you do not beat yourself up about how large this space is— you should dream big! We do not choose the cards that the universe decides to deal to us, and we have the ability to positively influence the outcome of decisions we have made. It is important that you treat your manifesto as a strategic documentation of how you plan to approach your goals. Take the time to write out the financial and time cost of what it would actually take to get there. If you like to have a daily latte, get your hair done once a month, or maybe consider taking a weekly hour-long class outside of the house, write down the full cost and assistance needed to factor that into your budget and scheduling. You might be surprised to find out that you are not that far away from your goals. Treat your assessments as the facts and figures that you need to nail down on your life's balance sheet. Remember, we are just putting everything down on paper to help you make sense of where you want to head—be sure to look out for signs of self-deprecation and reframe your perspective accordingly.

Set Clear Principles

The most essential part of any manifesto is its core values. Think about your principles—the nonnegotiable *musts* of your approach to life. What ethics do you believe motherhood must possess, unquestionably? What are the compulsory practices that you believe you must include in your documentation of your visionary life, and its set purposes?

To me, my most important core values are:

- practicing kindness
- practicing forgiveness
- treating others with respect
- putting in effort, regardless of what task it is that I am doing
- learning, whenever possible

Your principles are somewhat of the moral compass that you will shape your mothering manifesto with. You will need to streamline each of your topics with your principles, so make sure you cover everything—but try not to be too extensive. Essentially, your mom-ifesto should be something that you can read leisurely, whenever you want to feel motivated.

Boldly Proclaim

Now comes the fun part. Use your principles as a basis through which you will write about your topics. You can rephrase your aspirations, using your core values as the primary ingredients for your wording.

- In addressing my goal to take better care of myself, I could write:

"I will make an effort to be kind and compassionate toward myself, even when I do not meet my goals perfectly."

- In addressing my goal to be more patient with my children, I could write:
  "I will try my best to be patient with my children, treating them with the respect and kindness that they deserve."

There's no need to stick to a formula. You can be as straightforward or whimsical as you want to be. What matters is that you inspire yourself to work toward your goals. The language and approach that you attribute to your mom-ifesto depend on your individual tastes and outlook toward your life.

A friend of mine shared with me stories of a life as fantastical as she could manage it to be. I imagine her manifesto would include everything with her professions being statements like, "Trade your anxiety and fear of the world for bewilderment at its wonders." Another friend of mine in her own perfect way would have preferred statements like, "I will not let my ADHD stop me from accomplishing everything I planned today, even when there's no one here to judge me for it."

What motivates you is driven by the idiosyncratic notions that you have of yourself. Do not think too hard and ruin things. Have fun with your writing and be as ambitious as you desire!

Review

Go over what you've written. Take your words to be your mom-ifesto 'in the rough'. Remember, even though manifestoes conventionally work toward manifesting goals related, your review of your own manifesto should be authentic to the level of comfort and joy that you are able to receive through it.

Consider the following:

- Does your mom-ifesto allow you enough flexibility to not feel pressured by it?
- Does your mom-ifesto address your core values?
- You can review your goals by utilizing a mental role-play session. Imagine that you're not reading your own mom-ifesto, but the mom-ifesto of another woman with a similar mom resume. Factor in her hardships—the availability of help, the age of her children—and decide how achievable you find your aspirations to be. Scrap out anything too unrealistic, or particularly negative. In spite of everything, we tend to be more compassionate to other people than we are to ourselves—even if they're just like us.
- Have you addressed all aspects of your life that you had wanted to include in your mom-ifesto? Don't leave out the good stuff!

Write Concrete, Declarative Statements

Now that you've gotten the gist of what you want down on paper, you can work on summing up your statements in a short, and declarative manner. Remember to be bold about what you say about yourself. Modals like "will" and "always" can help bolden your statements. Work on summarizing your thoughts into a concise document that you will not have any trouble accessing whenever you feel the need to. Focus on getting your point across to yourself, rather than spending time on flashy statements, because the purpose of a manifesto is not to prove yourself to anyone but to create a memento that allows for self-inspiration when you are feeling low. Therefore, do not be afraid to make your mom-ifesto as personal, or as down-to-earth, as you need it to be.

In writing your mom-ifesto, you are essentially taking the first step into navigating your identity outside the boundaries of motherhood. By inquiring your innermost needs and desires, you are allowing for your spirit to be heard, without the backdrop of motherhood. Shaping an vision for yourself, without regards to a mother identity, establishes the level of detachment that you may want to practice with your children. As much as you love them, you have to realize and strive for your own goals. Your mom-ifesto will be your blueprint to a life of individuality, where you cannot use "the kids" as a suffix for your life aspirations. Allow your mind to register the fact that you have needs and ambitions that reach far outside the box that your domestic life may be putting you in. This stands to be the vital part of letting go of fear—both for yourself, and for your family.

Not So Hypothetical: Questions to Ask Yourself

- Why do you think mothers need to write their mom-ifestos?
- What part of the concept of a manifesto do you find beneficial to you, and your lifestyle?
- Can you think of someone you know personally who appears to have a life of balance and fulfillment? Based on their personality, what would their mom-ifesto look like?

CHAPTER 10

JOURNALING AS THERAPY

"Start writing, no matter what. The water does not flow until the faucet is turned on."

—LOUIS L'AMOUR

For as long as I can remember, I have always been that girl who best poured her heart out into a notebook. What started in elementary school (as a poor imitation of the diary-entry styled books with the heart lock that were all the rage at the time) grew to be a consuming habit (which I enjoyed) that would branch into the modes of song writing, poetry, and other forms of writing. Writing and song has always been the easiest way in which I learned to make sense of the world. Even for things as trivial as a schoolgirl crush, my first breakup, or the first time that I felt guilty for not taking care of a man—writing was always a vital part of the process by which I processed how I felt.

However, as attached as I was to personal writing, it took only 9 months, and a year of postpartum mayhem coupled with instability and social isolation to send me into writers block. The early days of motherhood, are as quintessential as they are colorful. It is hard to describe how acutely it first strikes you. Postpartum was present, and yet it was untouchable. It made me feel exhilarated, but it also terrified me. It made me fear what I might unleash on paper or in lyrics one day, had I simply let loose with my thoughts as I had always done but fuelled with my calculation for sleep as a negative equation. Another reason why postpartum was able to put my writing days to an unceremonious stop was that I had previously written as a way of preserving memories in the past. As magical as the process of bringing life into the world is, the magnanimity of the entire event doesn't always stick with you as enjoyable memorable moments emotionally and physically . At the time, I didn't want to remember some anxious distressing emotions for something as amazing as bringing human life into the world. So, I put them on the back burner.

It had been my first mom's support group that gave me a renewed interest in journaling. Most of the mothers in the group had a habit of essentially writing out journal entries as posts to each other on Facebook. This had me thinking. I thought about what it would be like to have a journal hour, where all of the mothers would sprawl on various sides of someone's living room and write. I went on a stationery frenzy and bought a ton of notebooks. To my surprise, most of the inventory I found marketed to women and mothers were not journals. Instead, most of the moms worked on mood trackers, gratitude, and to-do lists—little snippets of self-awareness that they could sprinkle into 10-minute sessions every day. I looked on Instagram for more. Some of the journal accounts I looked at looked like mine had always looked like—chicken scratch on paper. Others looked beautiful with Pinterest-worthy stickers, washi tape, and aesthetics that leveled the paper to collage-styled art.

Inspired by this, I made my first attempt (after many years of a writing hiatus) in this fashion. I bought fancy pens, and journaled my way through my first page of journaling. If putting pen to paper felt hard, I would use voice notes, or the notes section on my phone, constantly looking out for the gratitude, mental well-being, and sense of satisfaction that I found in my life. Soon enough, I was able to ease into a usual style of free thinking. What four long years off the page had taught me was that I was not writing to please anyone but myself. Writing anywhere could be a conveniently silent confidant or, as I would learn, a way of reinstating the power that I had over the events of my life.

Journaling can be a way in which you can show up for yourself, on a daily basis. The fact that you are in charge of what you say, and how you say it, means there's little to no pressure on your side. Journaling can help empower you, by raising the sense of compassion that you have for your life and reinvigorating your need to feel in charge of it. In my experience, journaling proved to be a cathartic way for me to come to terms with what I was feeling; it is where this book was born. Regardless of how you approach it, journaling can be a thoughtful self-actualization tool that may prove to be vital to leveling your emotions on a daily basis, and may someday benefit someone else too.

How Journaling Will Benefit You and Your Children

Journaling is considered to be one of the most efficient ways of helping people manage their stress and emotions. With the advent of its various forms, it can be a creative way for you to address different phases of your life. From pregnancy journals to memory books for your child's first year, the lined paper has evolved to a form that is able to cater to a wide range of the stages that you face in life. If you feel like you may benefit from templates and a preordained structure, you might enjoy using a bullet journal or a guided journal. On the other hand, if you prefer pouring your feelings into a free-writing session then go ahead!

The most important point of journaling, as a mode of therapy, is that you are authentic to both yourself and your needs as an individual. While my fear of my emotions had led me to a bad case of mental block, creative block, and writer's block in the past, my second blitz into the realm of journaling as a mom taught me that part of writing was facing my fears. I learned that as overwhelming as it was to sit with my mind as a mother in its sometimes worrisome presentment, the act of pouring my thoughts and emotions out of my mind and onto a page meant that I would have to face and make sense of my fears on a daily basis. This made me a braver person, and it taught me how to have compassion for myself even when I wasn't writing down my proudest achievements. Contrary to what I had once believed, rereading old logs that I had made during my daughter's first year fills me with a sense of pride for my strength. Looking back is always an interesting and enlightening experience, as it also adds perspective to the nature of our problems and the way they tend to affect us with time.

Furthermore, journaling can be used as a mode through which you can keep track of new habits that you want to include in your life and help you nourish more mindfulness into your lifestyle. For people on long-term medication for chronic illnesses, journaling can be a creative way of keeping tabs on new medications and changes in symptoms. Journaling has also been proven to help with memory issues. To those of us suffering from the effects of the mom brain, writing things down on a bullet list can help deal with the inevitable forgetfulness that managing a family comes with. Moreover, journaling doesn't have to be a *mom* thing either. You can make journal time a family activity, to stimulate more open conversation about feelings and emotions. Sit down with your family and keep your expectations low. Give them five minutes and let them approach their pages in their own ways. If your kids can't write yet, have them draw a picture of their day. Everyone has their own ways of expressing themselves. What your daughter best surmises with a doodle could amount to a page-long rant for you. You can use journaling as a way for your family to get in touch with their creativity while getting them into the habit of taking time to think about themselves and their personal well-being. The following section will cover some prompts to help you get started.

Journal Prompts to Get You Started

Prompt journaling is a popular way to get people attached to the page, as it removes the factor of having to think about what to write.

Listed below are a month's worth of journaling prompts just for you—feel free to customize them in accordance to your family dynamic:

- What are your goals for the next 30 days?
- What is the one thing you wish you had been told before you learned about it yourself?
- Write down three things you admire about yourself.
- What do you admire the most about your child?
- What is your proudest accomplishment?
- What is your best skill? Do you utilize this skill in your life?
- What are seven traits that you love about your partner?
- What things help you feel at peace with yourself?
- How do you practically improve how you parent?
- What is a gesture that you will do within 24 hours to show a loved one how much you cherish their presence in your life?
- What are the aspects of your kids' lives that make them the happiest?
- What is a gesture that you will extend toward your children in order to make them happy?
- How can you be a better friend? Include how you will bring these thoughts into action within a day.
- What are your worst fears?
- What is an aspect of your parenting style that you take pride in?
- What is an insecurity that you have about yourself, and how do you plan on confronting it?
- What is an insecurity that you have about your style of parenting, and how do you wish to deal with it?

- Write down an activity that you will partake in with your kids during the day that will make both you and your kids happy.
- What is a favorite childhood memory?
- Incorporate cherished games and childhood pastimes from when you were little into the lives of your children.
- Find a work-life balance.
- Considering spirituality and your family—what do you believe your children think of God? How do you want to manage the subject of religion with them?
- What are the most beautiful aspects of your life?
- What aspects of your life are you grateful for that others do not have the luxury of enjoying?
- In what ways can you make a stranger happy today?
- What behavioral traits of your child/ children tend to irritate you the most? How do you aim at processing these more patiently?
- What is a romantic activity that you used to do for fun before you had kids, and how do you plan on doing this again at present?
- What are some ambitions that you want to start working toward?
- Describe the degree of mindfulness that you incorporate in your lifestyle.

Not So Hypothetical: Questions to Ask Yourself

- What changes can you make to your lifestyle to ensure that you follow more mindful habits on a daily basis?
- How do you plan on using journaling as a form of therapy?

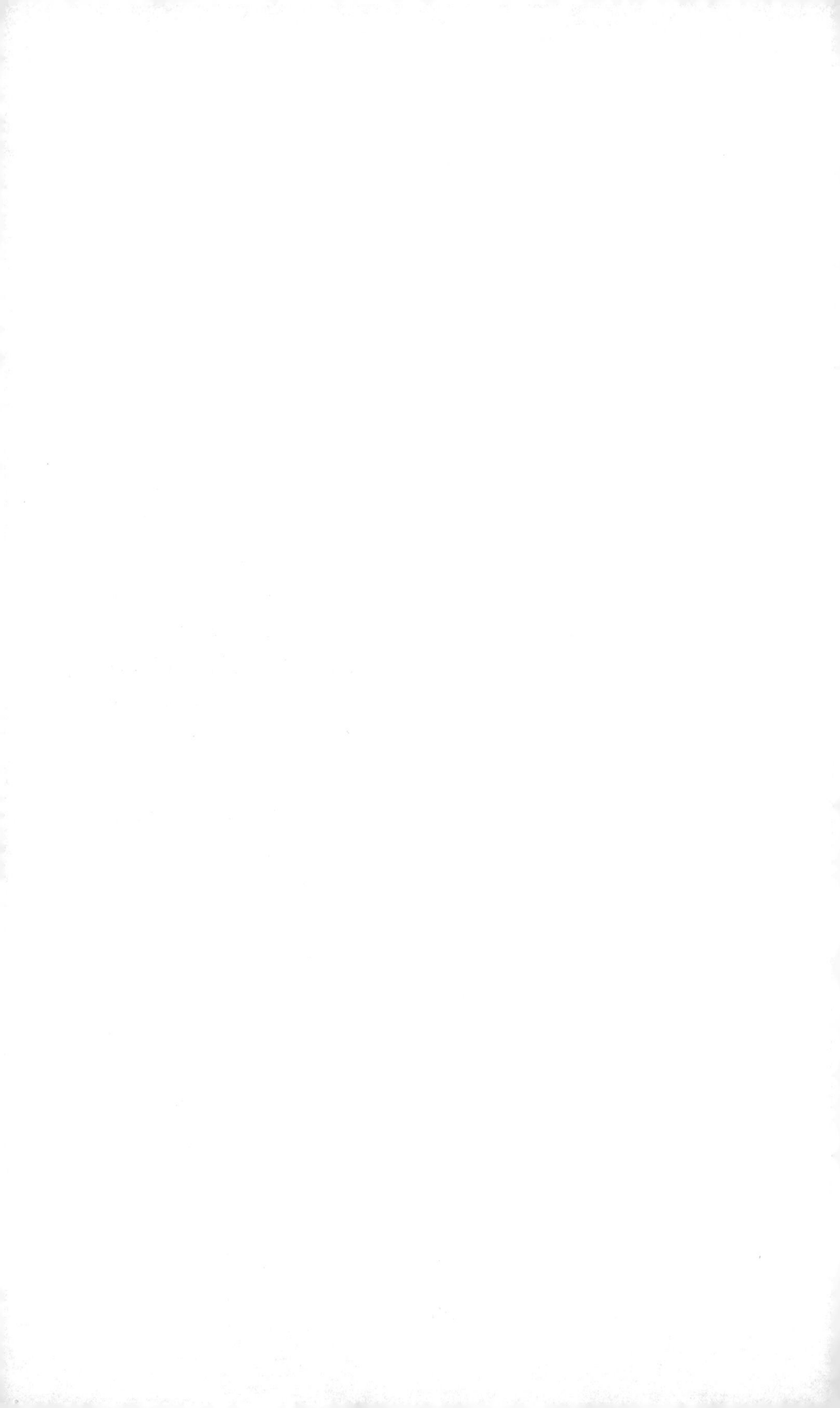

CONCLUSION

Looking back on my blue periods (to the many support groups of women who listened to me rant about women's rights and the many times I found myself on the phone with my best friend so far away. They take me back and I'm bewildered at the depth of knowledge that a woman's heart can carry), I tell myself that the journey is worth the difficult days. There's probably no need to describe them, because all of us with young children have felt them—the days we feel like our littles exist attached to our hips and screaming in our ears; the nights when the writing happens single-handedly, on the compact screen of a mobile phone while you nurse your little one to sleep. While it is true that there is still a long list of fundamental changes that need to be enacted constitutionally for true traditional feminism to be recognized on a universal front, the ideological gap that we have to penetrate through is trickier to catch and harder to tame.

Time has proven, on a repeated basis, that leaving women to expend their faculties entirely into their motherhood and with no compensation helps no one. We love our kids fiercely and unconditionally, with our entire soul and every beat of our hearts. However, what happens when they grow up, and don't need us as much? What happens when they have different needs than we do, or when they live life in a manner that is vitally eccentric to the one that we envisioned for them? They are their own person after all, not a piece of our property.

Investing your entire being into other people is not healthy— even if those people are your children. A mother is the only title which moulds to this identity and is not considered clinically unstable. You need space—to grow into yourself, and to allow your loved ones to experience life with a level of independence that exists outside your presence. In order to do this, you have to discover your voice of reason, and the aspirations that you hold for your life. Whether this means that you make the dreaded division of labor talk with your partner happen, or that you sit down beside a blank page and face the seeming vacancy of your heart, you need to get your act together.

As an individual, you owe yourself the right to your own joy. You owe yourself the pleasure of enjoying the gift of a comfortable motherhood—one that allows you enough space to breathe in and embrace its beauty. The beauty that was robbed from us by a structure without a sense of community, compensation for raising humans, and societal gaslighting. You need to be brave. If you've reached the end of this book, chances are that you've already been brave. It takes a certain level of courage to convince yourself to buy a *'self-help'* book, and *then* proceed to finish it. If you've already written your mom-ifesto, and spoken to your partner about the index card version of your chores, pat yourself on the back—you have successfully taken the leap.

Make sure to leave a review, if you've found any of these words to be helpful. On the other hand, if you are still resting between leaving what you've learned from the pages of this text and going for it with a heart-to-heart, don't beat yourself up. Change takes time. Don't let your mind push you to the back seat again. Start small. Tonight, attempt at your first conversation about your physical and mental load, or purchase your first prompt journal.

Remember Mama, you've brought life into this world, raised them this far, and done it all—you can do this!

LEAVE A REVIEW

Dear Mama,

This book took me two years to write and almost another two to publish. I fought many internal dialogues about who I was, if I was even worthy of being a mother, and I questioned so much of myself because of our system. If this book found itself to you and helped you in the way I intended it to, please share it with others. Share it with other moms, husbands, mothers-to-be, politicians (they need to hear it!), and anyone who should know that mothers are the mortar that holds humanity together, and that the lie we have been fed is complete BS and we know it.

Leaving an honest review not only helps me in my ambition to bring mothers to the front of the line and start of the discussion, but it also connects us all in the fight for a greater change that will make our lives and the lives of your children, and children's children better.

I would be incredibly thankful if I could take just 1 minute of your time to leave a rating and write a brief review on amazon even if it's just a sentence or two.

★★★★★

ACKNOWLEDGMENTS

This book started out as a bunch of notes on my iPhone that I wrote in the dark while nursing my firstborn, Hudson, and secondborn, Isabel, to sleep night after night... after night. Laying in the dark with them often felt connected and peaceful, but many nights there was so much happening in my mind that I had to get out of my head. If you didn't take so long to fall asleep, the pages of this book may not exist. So, thank you Hudson and Isabel for the struggles that felt so hard at the time– and thank you apple development team for the notes feature on my iPhone. I think I pushed the limits of what it was intended for. When I die, you may find that my iPhone notes are the thing that holds the strongest personal value to me in my will.

Mum, you are the single most amazing mother that I could have ever asked for. You sacrificed yourself in ways that I only now understand. I hope you know that your hard efforts and undeniable love will remain with me for the rest of my life. I am glad you found happiness with a partner after your days of parenting alone. I am the best version of myself because of you.

In addition, I want to thank all the mothers who were kind enough to share their candid stories with me–friends, acquaintances, and strangers on the internet all bound by motherhood. Your stories are gifts to the world and I hope that you write about them on your own one day. We all have a unique story to tell.

Finally, I want to thank Anna. There were months that went by where I experienced zero social interaction outside of my one-year-old, and occasionally my husband when he wasn't working. You called me and you always answered even though we were hundreds of miles away from each other. Our friendship is resilient.

REFERENCES

Adib, R. (2021, September 27). *5 balls of life: Coca-Cola's former CEO Brian Dyson's commencement speech on love, work, family and friendship.* Shine Coaching Barcelona. https://www.shinecoaching-barcelona.com/en/5-balls-of-life-brian-dyson-speech

Albom, M. (2014). *For One more day.* Hachette Books.

Anne Lamotte. (2015, April 8). I am going to be 61 years old in 48 hours. Wow. I thought I was only forty-seven [Post]. Facebook. https://www.facebook.com/AnneLamott/posts/662177577245222

Bureau, U. C. (2023, March 8). National Single Parent Day: March 21, 2023. Census.gov. https://www.census.gov/newsroom/stories/single-parent-day.html

Crilly, M. A., Bundred, P. E., Leckey, Li. C., & Johnstone, F. C. (2008, April 17). *Gender bias in the clinical management of women with angina: Another look at the yentl syndrome.* Journal of women's health (2002). https://pubmed.ncbi.nlm.nih.gov/18338964/

DeMarco, J. (2021, June 9). *53% of households are dual income — And that percentage has risen.* MagnifyMoney. https://www.magnifymoney.com/news/dual-income-households-study

Donovan, C. L. (2009). *The Ministry of Motherhood*. Peace in the Storm Pub.

Feder, B. (2019). *Just like your mother? Seven ways motherhood has changed (or not) in the last 25 years.* unfpa.org. https://www.unfpa.org/news/just-your-mother-seven-ways-motherhood-has-changed-or-not-last-25-years

Flagship programme: Making every woman and girl count. (n.d.). UN Women. https://www.unwomen.org/en/how-we-work/flagship-programmes/making-every-woman-and-girl-count

Gilman, C. P. (1892). *The yellow wallpaper*. The New England Magazine.

Goode, L. (2019, July 2). *Why everything from transit to iPhones is biased toward men.* Wired. https://www.wired.com/story/caroline-criado-perez-invisible-women

Grinspoon, P. (2022, May 4). *How to recognize and tame your cognitive distortions.* Harvard Health. https://www.health.harvard.edu/blog/how-to-recognize-and-tame-your-cognitive-distortions-202205042738

Howarth, J. (2023, January 9). *Time spent using smartphones (2023 statistics).* Exploding Topics. https://explodingtopics.com/blog/smartphone-usage-stats#top-smartphone-stats

Hutson, S. (2018, May 9). *How the role of being a mom has changed throughout history.* TheList.com. https://www.thelist.com/58638/how-role-mom-changed-throughout-history

Kay, K., & Shipman, C. (2014, April 15). *The confidence gap*. The Atlantic. https://www.theatlantic.com/magazine/archive/2014/05/the-confidence-gap/359815

Kirkova, D. (2013, September 17). *No wonder we feel exhausted! New parents lose 44 days of sleep in the first year of a child's life*. Mail Online. https://www.dailymail.co.uk/femail/article-2423615/New-parents-lose-44-days-sleep-year-childs-life.html

Kosin, J. (2019, January 6). *Glenn Close gives emotional, rousing Golden Globes acceptance speech*. Harper's BAZAAR. https://www.harpersbazaar.com/culture/film-tv/a25770458/glenn-close-golden-globes-acceptance-speech

Koziol, J. (2022, May 10). *America runs on mothers' sacrifice—and it's not OK*. Motherly. https://www.mother.ly/parenting/america-runs-on-mothers-sacrifice

Light, P. (2013, April 19). *Why 43% of women with children leave their jobs, and how to get them back*. The Atlantic. https://www.theatlantic.com/sexes/archive/2013/04/why-43-of-women-with-children-leave-their-jobs-and-how-to-get-them-back/275134

Matthews, M. (2016, May 8). *The Victorian baby: 19th century advice on motherhood and maternity*. Mimi Matthews. https://www.mimimatthews.com/2016/05/08/the-victorian-baby-19th-century-advice-on-motherhood-and-maternity

Meyer, J., & Lentz, P. (2006). *Battlefield of the mind winning the battle in Your mind*. Hachette Audio.

Nespor, C. (2014, June 25). *Debating women's "nervous temperament" in the 1890s*. Melnick Medical Museum. https://melnickmedicalmuseum.com/2014/06/25/womens-nervous-temperament

Rodsky, E. (2019). *Fair play: A game-changing solution for when you have too much to do (and more life to live)*. G. P. Putnam's Sons.

Samuel, S. (2019, November 22). *Women suffer needless pain because almost everything is designed for men*. Vox. https://www.vox.com/future-perfect/2019/4/17/18308466/invisible-women-pain-gender-data-gap-caroline-criado-perez

Single Mother Statistics (Updated 2022). (2021). Single Mother Guide. https://singlemotherguide.com/single-mother-statistics

Strayed, C. (2019). *Wild: From lost to found on the Pacific Crest Trail*. Alfred A. Knopf.

Tingley, L. (2021, November 14). *Being a mom isn't easy: 50 quotes for challenging days*. Simply Well Balanced. https://simply-well-balanced.com/being-a-mom-isnt-easy-quotes

Turlington Burns, C. (2011, November 17). *Sacrifices of motherhood*. HuffPost. https://www.huffpost.com/entry/maternal-mortality_b_858856

White, Tiara A. (2006, February). *Poem about difficulties being a mom, A mother's struggle*. Family Friend Poems. https://www.familyfriendpoems.com/poem/a-mothers-struggle

Winslow, L. (2016, October 1). *ESP between mothers and babies has been well documented - can we ...* Ezine Articles. https://ezinearticles.

com/?ESP-Between-Mothers-And-Babies-Has-Been-Well-Documented---Can-We-Duplicate-This-For-Others?&id=9603144

Zheng, X., Yuan, H., & Ni, C. (2022). Meta-research: How parenthood contributes to gender gaps in academia. *eLife*, 11. https://doi.org/10.7554/elife.78909

Made in the USA
Monee, IL
05 March 2024